Language Practices in Social W

Analysis of language and discourse in social sciences has become increasingly popular over the past thirty years. Only very recently has it been applied to the study of social work, despite the fact that communication and language are central to social work practice.

Language Practices in Social Work looks at how social workers, their clients and other professionals categorise and manage the problems of social work in ways which are rendered understandable, accountable and which justify professional intervention. Features include:

- studies of key sites of social work, such as home visits, case conferences, case notes, media reporting
- analysis of language and interaction used in typical case studies of everyday social work practice
- exploration of the ways in which professionals can examine their own practice and uncover the discursive, narrative and rhetorical methods that they use.

The purpose of this engaging study is to increase awareness of language and discourse in order to help develop better practices in social work. It is essential reading for social workers and will be of equal interest to discourse analysts in broader areas of social science.

Christopher Hall is Senior Research Fellow, Centre for Applied Childhood Studies, University of Huddersfield, UK.

Stef Slembrouck is Professor of English Linguistics and Discourse Analysis, University of Ghent, Belgium.

Srikant Sarangi is Professor of Language and Communication, and Director of the Health Communication Research Centre, Cardiff University, UK.

Language Practices in Social Work

Categorisation and accountability in child welfare

Christopher Hall, Stef Slembrouck and Srikant Sarangi

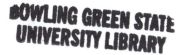

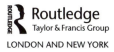
Routledge
Taylor & Francis Group

LONDON AND NEW YORK

First published 2006
by Routledge
2 Park Square, Milton Park, Abingdon, Oxon OX14 4RN

Simultaneously published in the USA and Canada
by Routledge
270 Madison Ave, New York, NY 10016

Routledge is an imprint of the Taylor & Francis Group

© 2006 Christopher Hall, Stef Slembrouck and Srikant Sarangi

Typeset in Goudy by
Keystroke, Jacaranda Lodge, Wolverhampton
Printed and bound in Great Britain by
The Cromwell Press, Trowbridge, Wiltshire

British Library Cataloguing in Publication Data
A catalogue record for this book is available from the British Library

Library of Congress Cataloguing in Publication Data
Hall, Christopher, Ph. D.
Language practices in social work : categorisation and accountability in
child welfare / Christopher Hall, Stef Slembrouck and Srikant Sarangi.
p. cm.
"Simultaneously published in the USA and Canada."
Includes bibliographical references and index.
ISBN 0-415-35687-3 (pbk) – ISBN 0-415-35686-5 (hardback).
1. Communication in social work. 2. Child welfare. 3. Interviewing.
4. Social service–Press coverage. 5. Discourse analysis–Social aspects.
I. Slembrouck, Stefaan, 1963– II. Sarangi, Srikant, 1956– III. Title.
HV29.7.H35 2005
362.7–dc22
2005016193

ISBN 10 0–415–35686–5   ISBN 13 9–780–415–35686–2 (Hbk)
ISBN 10 0–415–35687–3   ISBN 13 9–780–415–35687–9 (Pbk)

Contents

Acknowledgements

We would like to thank the many friends and colleagues who have supported our work over the last decade. We have been greatly encouraged by colleagues who see the potential of drawing on discursive and narrative methods for the study and development of social work. The DANASWAC-network (Discourse and Narrative Approaches to Social Work and Counselling) has become an important community for developing this kind of work and we thank all the members of this group. Particular thanks go to Susan White for reading and commenting on the manuscript and Nigel Parton for reminding us that the volume was still due on his shelf. We are also grateful to Chris Candlin who initially encouraged us to undertake a book on this topic. The data used in this book are drawn from various research projects and thanks to all the social workers and clients who have given their time to be interviewed and provide access. And finally many thanks to our families for their patience and encouragement.

In part, this book draws on previous work by the authors. In particular, Chapter 9 is a revised and extended version of 'Narrative transformation in child abuse reporting' which appeared in *Child Abuse Review* 6: 272–282 (1997). In addition some material appeared in earlier publications: part of Chapter 3 appeared in 'Moral construction in social work discourse', in B. Gunnarsson, P. Linell and B. Nordberg (eds) *The Construction of Professional Discourse*, London: Longman (1997), and Chapters 4 and 5 draw on 'The legitimation of the client and the profession in social work discourse', published in S. Sarangi and C. Roberts (eds.) *Talk, Work and the Institutional Order*, Berlin: Mouton de Gruyter (1999).

We are grateful to the following for permission to reproduce copyright material: the BBC for the extract from the programme *Someone to Watch Over Me*, broadcast on 14 December 2004 (Chapter 1); the Victoria Climbié Inquiry for the inquiry transcripts in Chapter 8; the *Guardian* for the report 'Death of child in care sparks inquiry call', 19 August 1989; the *Daily Mail* for the report 'Murdered girl was in danger all her life', 31 March 1990; the *Wandsworth Borough News* for the report 'Inquiry launched into child's murder', 6 April 1990 and *Community Care* for the reports 'Cuts contributed to child's death' and 'Action on child abuse', 28 June 1990 – all in Chapter 9.

1 Introduction

So it's mayhem up there

Social worker on the phone

Social worker: Believe it or not we've actually got four child protections all on intensive care. So it's mayhem up there. So the consultant hasn't yet I mean he said he'll come back to me with more information but I mean I think it is extremely questionable if this child will survive. They are clear that at this stage it is a child protection referral.

This is the opening of a television programme *Someone to watch over me* broadcast on the BBC in December 2004. It was the last in a series of six programmes about social workers in Bristol in the UK during 2003. Each programme followed how two or three social workers managed their work with children and families, with clips from meetings with other professionals and parents, telephone conversations and shots to camera. They aimed to display the crises and tragedies which are the daily dilemmas of social workers. The cases were all very serious with children injured, at risk, in care and, in this case, the baby had serious brain injuries. After this opening we become witness to various meetings and commentary from professionals which took place in the hospital, relating to one of the four cases, a baby with severe brain damage.

Meeting between social worker and doctors

Doctor: Now this little one is 6 months old whilst feeding become very floppy and stopped breathing.

Social worker: In Dad's care?

Doctor: I haven't got that yet ehm and a CT scan was done which showed left temporo-parietal haemorrhages and inter-hemispheric fissural haemorrhages. During the transfer to Bristol both pupils became fixed and dilated and a repeat CT scan showed generalised brain oedema with complete loss of all ventricles and this morning the child is having a lot of very abnormal movements. The radiologist has the impression from the CT scans that this is not survivable ehm appearance.

Doctor 2: Ok yeah. Catastrophic brain trauma isn't it ehm. I mean at some point we are going to need to let them know that the police will need to talk to them and social services.

Social worker: And check basics like are there any other children.

Having heard this serious diagnosis, the professionals meet to plan the next stage.

Meeting in social work office

Social worker: The parents are here. They are stressed. They don't know there is any query on the explanation they have given that he choked and became floppy.

Team manager: That's what they think. That's what. That's their.

Social worker: At the moment.

Doctor: We need to go and talk to these parents and broach the child protection issues. Following I think that we'll try and examine him.

Team manager (writing notes): So see parents, inform police and record plan in the medical notes about in the event of death.

Doctor: It's potentially. If he does die, I mean, we are dealing with a murder.

The father denies that he harmed his son and has told the social worker that the baby choked while he was feeding him. The baby's mother is standing by him. The family live some distance from the hospital and the social worker's priority is to inform their local police of the latest developments.

Commentary to camera

Social worker: It's really sad. My job in this kind of circumstance is to ascertain facts and get an account from the parents and explain to them what's happening.

Social worker on the phone to police

Social worker: His injuries are consistent with being shaken they are . . . we're very unlikely to get any other medical explanation but they are still obviously . . . checking everything they've got. But whether he started coughing and Dad panicked and shook him as part of trying to deal with that situation he started choking. Or whether he was shaken and that led to a choking we don't we don't know. I hear what you are saying you're dealing with a potential murder inquiry and all the rest of it but I can just say that these are coming across as ehm distraught parents.

(We don't hear the response from the police)

Social worker: Alright. Yeah yeah yeah. (sigh) I know it's the wrong time of night for me to do this but can I play devil's advocate? Can we keep this Dad up here ehm even if you have to arrest up here and can you interview him up here. Alright? Speak to you tomorrow. Bye bye.

(Social worker puts down the phone)

Team manager: Who was that?

Social worker: Detective Inspector.

Team manager: Right I think I've got the gist of all that.

Social worker: Bollocks.

Team manager: Are they pushing?

Social worker: His boss is saying 'arrest and bring him back to Cornwall'.

Team manager: No no no no no.

Social worker: Well. You heard my no no no no and I said well there's no point in my saying no no no no even though in my head I'm going no no no no no and that's why you heard me say 'these are just distressed parents'. Is there any way if you have absolutely got to arrest him, is there any way of doing it in Bristol?

The social worker clarifies how she is trying to communicate her point of view to the police.

Commentary to camera

Social worker: Because they didn't know anything about the case they seemed to spend a large part of the day going 'this is really serious this is a shaken baby' just getting it through. And they were going 'yeah yeah but we need more medical information' and just try to make sure that everybody had got the severity of the situation. And now I'm like 'hang on, why do you need to get up here and arrest him tonight?' And you know maybe this chap has murdered him and maybe I'm absolutely wrong in saying that but you've got parents that are extremely distressed. He was coming across as a doting dad who had been really scared and if he . . . The majority of times that babies and children are shaken parents do not plan to do it and they're not parents that don't care. They are parents that love their babies that go beyond it. Now that doesn't mean it's right. It doesn't mean you can allow that child to stay there. You've got to take all the action but it's not some cold calculating monster. It's a loving parent.

Team manager: I've seen them come up to the ward and take parents off before now. And we've fought very hard for that not to happen.

The police are going ahead with the arrest.

Commentary to camera

Social worker: I can't get away from the belief that whatever political body it is in government if they really cared about vulnerable people in society they would put more resources into it. Because they know they know how many families we are working with you know nationally. They know what work we are doing. If they run it so that people have so many cases and are continually working to their absolute maximum capacity and beyond because there aren't enough staff and there aren't enough resources, then they should take some responsibility for when things go wrong.

The police go ahead with the arrest in the hospital and take the father away to his home area, some 200 miles away. The social workers and the police meet.

Meeting with police

Team manager: Why did he have to go down under the circumstances?
Police: I can't really comment on that. It's a decision made by my D[etective] I[nspector].
Team manager: Fine. Ok.
Social worker: At the risk of being . . . If we can work out why (inaudible) If we can just get him back.

Team manager: I've got to just go and fax something on another case that we've got to go in and remove a baby . . . I'll just find out what I've done with the papers.

Police (on the phone to his superior): Hello Tom, it's Harry. Have you received a fax that's come through there? It's a letter written by the consultant ehm who is in charge of the case this morning. Well, ehm it's got, well, I'll read it to you with regards to this patient. 'It is imperative that this father be transported to the Bristol Children's Hospital immediately.'

Social worker on the phone

Social worker: They arrested him in front of other parents in our parents room huhh and ehm he went for . . . That was by Bristol Police on the instruction from Cornwall. And then he was taken down to Cornwall and we've spent the morning frantically trying to get him back.

Planning in social work office

Social worker: What I need to do is ask the admin to cancel Karin. Are you ok? Alright? (Social worker puts an arm on the team manager's shoulder)

Team manager: Yeah. I've just got so much on.

Social worker: Don't worry. Karin we are alright. We'll get through today. I'm just going to ask admin to cancel appointments. We'll get through today.

Team manager: But what about?

Social worker: And then we'll do tomorrow.

The next day, social workers meet with the police to present the evidence.

Meeting with police

Social worker: We met with the parents yesterday. 5pm. Dad felt he was starting to be hungry started feeding him. I don't know what he was feeding. He took he estimates about 10 mouthfuls of food and then he closed his mouth.

Police (takes notes): 10 mouthfuls of unknown food.

Social worker: Yeah and then he started coughing. He opened his mouth during this and he could see that there was food in his mouth so he said that he took the spoon and tried to gently scrape the food from around his mouth. He continued to cough ehm and was choking. He was really distressed. He was panicking. He began to panic at that point. He put him on his shoulder and had been ehm patting his back.

Police: Did he say how many times he patted his back?

Social worker: No. And he went limp and remained limp throughout. He dialled 999. He then heard the sirens and ran out. He was very clear in saying that he had not shaken him at all.

Police: He actually said that, did he?

Social worker: Yes.

Police: Who informed them this last evening. There were the fact that there were the suspicious nature of the injuries.

Social worker: They were informed yesterday evening.

Police: Yesterday evening.

Social worker: That the injuries were consistent with him being shaken.

Police: Ok.

Social worker: They answered everything they were asked. He understood that we needed to do our jobs but they felt that they were being accused and the fact that it was such a serious and distressing time for them.

Team manager: I mean. Is it not inhuman to let him see his child through his life and then, you know, dig in.

Police 2: Obviously that's a decision that we didn't make.

Social worker: No.

Police 2: That's the problem. It's going to be 'don't shoot the messenger' because people other than us our managers made the decision.

Team manager: Yes, I appreciate that.

Social worker: I don't understand why he had to be taken back to Cornwall.

Police: If we were to charge with any offences, they would have to go to court in our police area.

Team manager: I mean down that motorway, I mean it's a good three three hours.

Police: Easily, easily three hours.

Commentary to camera

Social worker: This family may feel that they spoke to myself and the doctor and as a result of that he's now been arrested and they may they may feel that he was honest with us that he was open with us and look what's happened. And they may feel that to take him away from their son, from his partner, at this time is just unbelievably uncaring. If his son dies, not to have the option to be there, is is a huge thing.

Some time later that week, the social worker learns that the baby has died. His father was brought back to hospital in time. Eight months later all charges against him were dropped. The parents are planning to lodge a formal complaint against the police. The case has prompted the police to change their arrest procedures. At the end of the week, the social worker is exhausted.

Commentary to camera

Social worker: It's just been such a gawd awful week really and what I set out to do on Monday morning it's now half past three on Friday afternoon I'm still nowhere near doing it. One child's died. One child got appalling scans and is in another hospital. And the third one is you know very uncertain prognosis. And I've just got work coming out of my ears and I don't know where to start. (sigh) There are too many too many balls plates, in the air and if I think, if I think about each individual plate, I kind of know what I'm juggling but I can't do all the plates. If I dropped one of the plates, badly, and I think I'd be held squarely responsible for that. And I think the fact that you are juggling all the other plates won't count for a lot because you should have picked up on the plate you just dropped.

The social worker carried on in the children's hospital for another six months. After that she went on long-term sick leave.

Commentary to camera

Social worker: I woke up one morning and I felt numb and emotionally dead inside and all of a sudden things that were normal parts of my life became impossible. What's surprised me really was talking to colleagues and friends in social work. Everybody I know has either been through it or know someone who has been through it in some form or another and I think it's what people term as burn out.

Why is she in this line of work?

Social worker: For me motivation is supporting families people through a time of crisis. That could happen to me could happen to anyone. We're trying to do our best for families. I'm still feeling numb so that tells me I got a way to go yet but I'm getting there and I will go back.

The case described in this programme highlights many of the pressures, demands and dilemmas of contemporary social work with children and families. Social workers are involved in tragic family circumstances on a daily basis, although thankfully the death of children remains relatively rare (in 2002 and 2003, 99 children were killed in England and Wales, Home Office, 2004). They make contact with parents and children when extremes of distress and emotion are uppermost, and are frequently the target of violent and threatening behaviour – one of the other social workers in the series was seriously assaulted and another threatened with a knife.

Social workers are constantly balancing competing demands, risks and responses – children's versus parents' needs, caring versus confrontational stances, immediate versus measured reactions. As the series producer says on the website (Johnson 2004):

The series explores the complex relationship between the British public and the social services – on the one hand, social workers are condemned for repeatedly getting it wrong and not doing enough, whilst on the other, people like to deride 'busy body' social workers for interfering.

Or as it is sometimes put, they are 'damned if they do, and damned if they don't'.

They cannot work in isolation and inevitably communicate and collaborate with other professionals – in this case, doctors, the police, but also teachers, nurses, youth workers, health visitors, housing officials, psychologists, foster parents, residential workers, etc. Whilst often such multi-professional action works well, sometimes other professionals do not share the same sensibilities about what is appropriate action, and there are conflicts and compromises.

There is a shortage of resources with staff overworked and stressed. In the Victoria Climbié Inquiry (2001–2002) there was criticism that the main social worker had 19 rather than 12 cases – in this programme one of the social workers had 43 cases. At one point during the filming, one of the emergency duty teams had nearly 40 per cent of posts vacant, and a quarter of those off sick were off with stress-related long-term sickness. Yet, it seems that successive governments have chosen to criticise, sometimes malign, social work rather than see it is a central part of the welfare network, with threats to undermine their status or remove responsibilities. Only in recent years has professional registration and financial support for training begun, much later than, for example, for nurses or teachers.

Given the pressures, successes will always be overshadowed by failures. As the social worker demonstrated with her metaphor of 'plates in the air', if one is dropped the struggle to keep up the others will not be seen as mitigation. And when mistakes are made, people's lives can be dramatically affected – children are hurt and worse, families are split up, children's development is disrupted.

For the social workers themselves their close involvement with children and families means they are intimately involved in successes and failures. When things go well with families able to care for their children without further concerns or children rescued from abusive homes, then the rewards are high, although rarely acknowledged. When things go wrong and interventions do not protect children, social workers can take failure personally with tears and self-doubt and, for some, burn out.

How then can commentators react? The programme makers of the BBC series were sympathetic. The social workers' point of view was given prominence and rarely challenged by other voices. Statements like 'I don't trust social workers' by some parents were given little credence when set against some of their actions. Whilst the programme's coverage was broadly supportive, given substantial filming over 15 months, and dramatically displayed some of the dilemmas, inevitably only certain aspects could be portrayed. Viewers do not know what was edited out or what were the consequences of subtle splicing. Perhaps the main message of the programme was that social workers are more competent and less authoritarian than is commonly portrayed in the media and that they are seriously under-resourced and under-supported.

However, for academic commentators this is not enough. We have a more considered goal, even a scientific responsibility to comment on social work. Unlike TV programme makers, we are less able to display ideas by providing dramatic portrayals; instead, we are seen as experts and expected to provide answers to problems.

Evidence-based approaches

One critical response to routine practice by academics and others has been to suggest that if only social workers examined research on child development, parenting and social work interventions, they would be guided by evidence and make better decisions, and risks to children would be diminished. It suggests that the dilemmas that social workers face can be assessed and certain attributes of people and events identified. Such assessments can then be set against rigorous research evidence of similar people and events and what happened. Consequently, interventions are prescribed in line with research evidence and the outcomes measured. This is often referred to as 'evidence-based practice'. Such an approach has gathered widespread support amongst some academics and fits well with government attempts to measure performance and regulate practice.

There is considerable debate about the efficacy of evidence-based practice and it is not appropriate to review the positions of proponents and critics here (see for example Ixer 1999; Sheldon 2001; Taylor and White 2002; Webb 2001). However, the case above highlights some of the difficulties which might be encountered when attempting to apply a rigid version of evidence-based practice to real life situations. First, the evidence of whether the baby had been intentionally killed is not clear when the social worker had to take action on the case. Although the medical evidence was considered to be 'consistent' with the baby having been shaken, issues of culpability are much more complex. The x-rays only tell part of the story since the intentions, motives and state of mind of the father would require detailed scrutiny before blame could be apportioned. Medical and legal argument would take several months for these issues to be resolved during which time the social worker had to act. Second, assessment and action was multi-professional and the social worker has to work with the practices and assessments of other professionals. Here the actions of the police were at odds with the social workers' view of appropriate responses. They restricted what social workers could do. Assessments and action would necessarily involve negotiations with other professionals and probably parents rather than merely implementing decisions based on evidence and analysis. In the context of joint decision-making, emergency responses and uncertain evidence, it is hard to see how evidence-based practice could replace what has been dismissed as 'opinion-based decision-making' (Webb 2001:62).

To highlight the problems of rigid adherence to evidence-based practice does not however suggest that professional practice can be characterised as ad hoc or irrational. It suggests that what actually happens in the practice of everyday professional work might be attempts at rational decision-making but set within competing demands of managing uncertainties, negotiations with others and getting by with initial formulations of people and events, all of which takes place within contexts of political imperatives, policy formats and resource constraints. As Cicourel (1976: 47) notes, even the early proponents of rational decision-making theory acknowledged that 'rationality is approachable but not achievable'.

Reflective approaches

Whilst not necessarily in direct opposition to evidence-based practice, an alternative response to improve professional work has been termed 'reflective practice' and 'critical reflection'. This approach sees social work practice as characterised by uncertainty and rarely susceptible to the rational process of unambiguous evidence and clear choices. Instead, social workers are confronted with the problems of distressed people in complicated and unpredictable situations. Not only are families' situations unique and not easily equated with the neat categories of research findings, social workers do not merely implement technical strategies. How they understand a family situation and how they carry out their work are a product of a variety of extraneous influences – for example, the workers' experience and training, their personal and professional values, the remit and culture of their agency. Furthermore, policies and practices which promote empowerment or partnership in decision-making mean negotiation. Seeking agreements with families and other parties place further restrictions on the implementation of rational methods.

In contrast to evidence-based approaches, reflective practice does not see such restrictions on the application of rational methods as a problem but as an opportunity for critical appraisal and professional development. Especially when faced with a lack of clear evidence, the reflective practitioner relies on intuitive action, making decisions based on experience and juggling often conflicting propositions. Rather than relying on external formal methods of analysis, practitioners are encouraged to make spaces to reflect on their practice and examine the dilemmas and concerns, with the help of colleagues or supervisors. In this way, practitioners are seen as gaining insights into how they carry out their work and are encouraged to challenge what Wilkinson (1999: 36) calls 'the constraints of habituated thoughts and processes'.

Again there are criticisms of such approaches; in particular that such reflection is merely 'benign introspection' (Woolgar 1988, quoted in White and Stancombe 2003: 19), looking inwards rather than engaging with the others. Furthermore, by promoting intuitive practice and critical reflection, the resulting formulation is set up as in some way superior to other versions, and as such unavailable to examination or challenge (Taylor and White 2000: 193). At the same time, the client's version may be marginalised since the professional might assert, after careful reflection, they are able to speak on behalf of the client (Taylor 2003: 249).

In the case above, we see even at the earliest stage of contact how the social worker is engaged in creating intuitive formulations of the father. She recognises that there are alternative versions of what actually happened and how his culpability will be examined as more evidence becomes available. However, her initial formulation of the case includes assessment of the parents' capacities, 'a doting dad'. Such a characterisation is a very strong formulation in the circumstances with little evidence of what happened. The father is portrayed as a 'loving parent' and contrasted with 'a cold calculating monster'. Such a formulation might have been based on a variety of instance observations and experience of similar cases – parents who shake their children don't often mean to do it and these particular parents appear 'distraught'. Whilst such initial formulations may be revised in response to new evidence, they are strong instant characterisations which may be hard to challenge.

Moreover, it can be questioned whether such a formulation is only a product of the workers' individual assessment of the father's character. The characterisation is produced in a series of encounters with the others, notably the police, and supported by the team manager. In particular the social worker can be seen using the formulation to counter what are seen as callous arrest procedures. The formulation also draws on versions of proper procedure when families are facing the death of their child. So the formulation might not be more than intuitive practice but have significant strategic functions to manage the interactions with other professionals.

The turn to language and enhancing social work

The approach taken in this book will step back from both evidence-based and reflective approaches to professional practice. Our suggestion is that the study of how social workers carry out their work will benefit from the detailed study of mundane activities and this entails the study of language use and interaction. One could use the description here: practice is mediated by language and interaction. By language use we mean all forms of spoken and written communication and by interaction we mean all encounters between social workers, clients and others where social work is practised.

We do not challenge the importance of gathering evidence, or the need for social workers to consider carefully the various contexts in which they work with children and families. However, we want to retreat from offering solutions and instead direct attention to observing some of the ways in which professional practice actually takes place. We hope to describe and illuminate the practice of social work rather than promote or undermine it.

Whilst social workers gather evidence, assess parents' capacities and risks to children, and consider their own feelings, all such ambitions take place in mundane activities which remain largely unexplored in the discussions about what social workers do. Daily work for social workers involves making phone calls, writing reports, talking to clients, colleagues and other professionals, holding meetings. Such activities involve talking, writing, interacting and negotiating with others. These mundane features of daily professional life are not insignificant processes which merely operationalise, facilitate or frustrate evidence-based practice or critical reflection. On the contrary, the objectives of social work can only be realised through such mundane activities and these practices do not just have an influence on social work, they constitute it, they bring it into existence.

A much quoted illustration of these different positions about the nature of social reality is provided by Sarbin and Kituse (1994: 1):

> Three baseball umpires are reflecting on their professional practice of calling balls and strikes. The first, a self-confident realist says, 'I call 'em the way they are,' to which the second who leans toward phenomenological analysis says, 'I call 'em as I see 'em', and the third closes the discussion with 'They ain't nothin' until I call 'em.'

For the third umpire, 'the constructionist umpire', it is only by his action that the entity, in this case the ball, is brought into existence and assigned meaning and significance. Similarly for the social worker above, it is only when she formulates a description of the father as a 'doting dad' that she produces a version of the father from the point of view of the child protection investigation and in doing so makes important inferences about who is to blame, to what extent and what should happen next. This is not to suggest that the father (or the ball) did not exist before the social worker's (or umpire's) intervention. However, the everyday assessments and actions of the professionals make the father (and the ball) real for the task at hand. Such assessments and actions take place in particular settings, with constraints, required routines and established traditions with various audiences monitoring the efficacy of the professional practice.

This tradition of seeing language and interaction as constructing and constituting social reality has a long history and has influenced considerable analysis and research of professional practice in recent years. Heath and Hindmarsh (2002: 99) note the importance of early ethnographic studies of organisations (e.g. Hughes 1958) in which the study of social interaction was central:

> Social interaction lies at the heart of organisational life. It is through social interaction that organisations emerge and are sustained; it is a consequence of social interaction that people develop routines, strategies, practices and procedures, and it is by virtue of social interaction that clients receive, and perceive, goods and services in ways defined by the organisations and its occupation[s].

Similarly Gunnarsson *et al.* (1997: 1) note the importance of discourse in the study of professional practice:

> Written texts, spoken discourse and various forms of non-verbal communication have all played essential parts in the historical creation of professional practices and they continuously contribute to the gradual reproduction and reshaping of these practices. Though the processes are as old as the professions, the interest in the understanding of the dynamics of professional discourse is quite new and growing among researchers as well as practitioners.

This approach to analysis has been described as concerned with the 'seen but unnoticeable' features of everyday practice (Garfinkel 1967: 180). It examines how participants in conversation and writing create understandings, manage disputes, reach agreements and silence others in ways which they may well be unaware of. Through the use of persuasive verbal practices, speakers create competing versions of the world which they defend in encounters with others. Unfortunately there are few approaches to the study of social work in comparison with the work on, for example, doctor–patient communication or classroom interaction (notable exceptions include Hall 1997; Hall *et al.* 1997a, 1997b; Hall *et al.* 1999a, 1999b; Hall *et al.* 2003a; Hall and Slembrouck 2001; Dingwall *et al.* 1983; Floersch 2002; Jokinen *et al.* 1999; de Montigny 1995; Parton *et al.* 1997; Sarangi 1998a; Seltzer *et al.* 2001; Slembrouck 2003, 2004, 2005; Taylor and White 2000; White and Stancombe 2003).

What marks the writers referred to above is both a commitment to the study of language and interaction and a recognition of the importance of the practice of social work. Our work does not rely on the promotion of social work values and philosophies of practice. Nor do we embrace explanations which ignore issues that are of concern to the profession. For instance, we accept that the concept of parental participation is a social work principle, and carry out research oriented to language use and interaction concentrating on its realisation in everyday encounters (Hall and Slembrouck 2001). A social work academic might promote the principle without giving sufficient credence to everyday practice. A language researcher might see the principle as being of little concern, choosing instead to examine the micro-interactional dynamics as an end in itself. For us, 'micro-interaction' is 'parental participation'. In the case of the present book, this dual orientation is reflected in the personal biographies of the authors and the nature of their joint authorship. One author has long experience as a practitioner and researcher of social work policy and practice. The other two authors have a long interest in the discursive study of various professions and the working of institutions and organisations. Concepts of sympathetic involvement and distanced observation have been central to the research. This has been a dynamic process, in which each author has often embraced the other's point of view.

This book will build on these approaches to the study of social work language and interaction. The two key theoretical concepts, categorisation and accountability, will underpin the analysis and are explored in Chapter 2. The former is concerned with how professionals and clients manage information in order to produce ways of understanding family problems and to direct their action. The latter concept of accountability considers the way speakers and writers monitor their talk and text in order to display themselves as competent, authoritative and trustworthy.

The substantive chapters are divided into two sections. The first section is concerned with the talk and writing of the social workers themselves – interviews, meetings, home visits, case notes. The second section concerns others talking or writing about social workers – clients, lawyers, journalists. Each chapter will concentrate on the analysis of one or two cases, although others will be discussed through cross-references from other relevant studies. Each chapter will introduce the topic in terms of professional concerns and at the end will examine how far the analysis has enabled the professional problem to be explored.

Chapter 3 draws on data from two interviews in which social workers are asked to explain (and thereby justify) their work with particular families as part of a policy review. The central issue here is: how social workers produce explanations of their work which is heard as professionally justified. Here we illustrate how social workers produce stories to explain their assessments and actions. It focuses not only on the sequential structures of storytelling but develops the notions of making accountable decisions, establishing and maintaining client categories, and a concern with risk management and the allocation of responsibility and blame.

Much of social work is carried out in meetings involving co-professionals and the analysis in Chapter 4 is based on the transcription of a child protection conference. There has been a concern that discussion in case conferences is influenced by the internal dynamics of the meeting. Our analysis demonstrates how professionals seek to cooperate with one another in constructing shared versions of the moral character of the parents. In this case, the mother is discussed in terms which establish her love and care but also her deficiencies and hence the dangers to her children. The nature of description and evaluation in the case conference is organised around depicting the mother's character rather than focusing on the nature of the abuse that the children face.

The data in Chapter 5 is a home visit by a social worker to a mother whose daughter has been abused by her husband. In line with the literature, which notes that notions of the roles of client and social worker are vague, we explore how such statuses are negotiated in the interview. How does the mother depict herself as a responsible mother but needy client and how does the social worker construct a legitimate professional role in this case? In this setting, the categories of social worker and client are less explicitly identified, so participants have to reach agreement through hints and positioning which illustrate rather than define roles and statuses.

Case notes and client records are an important site of professional work and are explored in Chapter 6. They are institutional requirements, but generally constitute a professional resource as what goes into case notes is a professional judgement. They offer a window on the inside of professional activities, although it is important to recognise that case notes need to be interpreted in terms of their intended audience, often fellow professionals. The analysis will focus on aspects of recontextualisation, i.e., how talk with fellow professionals, clients, etc., is translated into text and acquires the status of institutional reality. In other words, case records become cases by mediating between alternative accounts/categorisations and have the potential to influence future action.

In more than one respect Chapter 7 offers a mirror image of the policy interview chapter. It draws on an extended interview which one of the researchers had with a parent of an infant in public care. It raises the question of an alternative account centred on the client's experiences at the receiving end of social work practice, with the analysis focusing on parents' own explanations, their positioning vis-à-vis institutional intervention, diagnoses and categories, and the rhetorical figures used to redeem their own parenthood. There is also an issue of power here: when can a client say 'I don't want this intervention any more', especially when they themselves initiated the contact with the social services?

Social work often attracts public scrutiny following high profile cases. The Victoria Climbié Inquiry (2003) has made publicly available a large amount of data on the identification of child abuse and the justification of professional practice. Chapter 8 analyses the cross-examination by the inquiry barrister of two of the social workers involved in the case. It considers the ways in which the barrister and social worker construct and manage how Victoria's case was seen as a child protection or family support case. What is at stake is how professional action which went wrong can be justified or blamed.

Since the 1970s, a series of high profile child abuse cases have aroused widespread media coverage and criticism of social work. Social workers often feel that this media scrutiny has been unduly critical of their work and has undermined their status. However, the coverage has not always been uniform, with a wide range of factors determining how a case is reported. Chapter 9 looks at one of the lower profile cases, Stephanie Fox in 1990. It follows the reporting at different stages of the process – arrest, prosecution, inquiry findings, and in different types of media – national, local and professional press.

The final chapter draws together the central themes of the book. It considers how the concepts of accountability and categorisation can contribute to professional studies more generally. In particular, it discusses what discourse/narrative analysis has to offer to social workers in terms of analysing their work practices and how it contributes to reflexive and social constructionist approaches to social work.

2 Categorisation and accountability in professional texts and talk

Introduction

In this chapter we outline some of the theoretical formulations which underpin the analysis of professional discourse and which shape our investigation of social work text and talk. In particular we discuss the concepts of accountability and categorisation.

Our approach is discourse analytic. This means that we wish to foreground how professional processes are constructed in everyday activity and how they depend on communicative processes. It is suggested that any claims to truth by social workers, clients or other professionals have to be acted out in professional settings for them to matter. Facts, opinions and assessments have to be worked on and worked up in talk or in writing. The professional and the client will gather pieces of information and comment to support their version of events and to persuade others of its veracity. Such performances in meetings, interviews or in writing will require a range of persuasive and interactional devices (e.g. the way professionals in case conferences struggle to present their version of the case – see Chapter 4).

Nor can facts and opinion be separated from their presentation. To say that a child is being abused will be affected by who is making the claim (for example a neighbour or paediatrician), where the claim is made (in the office or at court), what are the consequences of the claim (will the child will be removed or the family offered support), or who is listening (the police or a research interviewer).

It is suggested then that the everyday processes of social work inevitably involve setting in motion processes which aim to produce assessments of what type of case this is or what is going on here. Furthermore, such activities will involve paying attention to concerns about how such assessments are presented and justified. Such processes can be explored in terms of key themes from discourse theory and research: categorisation and accountability. Accountability refers to the way in which assessments and action are justified in terms appropriate to contexts and events. For example, a description of a 'failure-to-thrive' case displays the opinions of doctors and records of weight loss (Hall *et al.* 1997a). Categorisation involves a set of processes which result in facts, opinions or circumstances being established as one type or category rather than another; for example, this is a case of 'failure-to-thrive', not delayed development (Hall 1997: 93). Whereas for social workers categories are a means to an end (e.g. to set in motion an effective intervention or treatment), we are mainly interested in how categories come about and the kind of work that needs to be done to establish, define, defend, refute, etc. them. As Shotter (1993: 9) puts it, 'what matters is not so much the conclusions arrived at as the terms within which arguments are conducted'. In making claims that a particular category is appropriate, the actor will deploy a set of textual and verbal devices to justify that the claim is true and that they demonstrate that s/he can be held accountable for the claim in terms appropriate to the context.

It is not our aim to undermine or criticise professional processes on the basis of ideas about social work practice and theory. As Silverman says (1997: 35), 'my preference is not to criticise professionals but to understand the logic of their work'. We prefer to see categorisation and accountability as interactional and rhetorical processes which can be observed in the everyday talk and writing of professionals. Our analysis does not seek to comment on the accuracy of the categorisation process but on how it takes place and its consequences. How professionals talk and categorise families has significant effects on what happens to them. Neither is there an assessment made of the success of the accounting performances; instead, our aim is to investigate how it is achieved with particular effects.

Accountability, rhetoric and moral concerns

While the accountability of the professional is often talked of in terms of overall responsibilities enshrined in law or in professional codes of practice, in everyday interaction speakers are constantly attending to how their speech renders their actions accountable. There are many facets to professional accountability: accountability as defined legally, as practised intra-professionally, as interpreted by the media or by the public more generally, etc. For instance, in a public inquiry into a child death the concern is with identifying how far professionals lived up to the responsibilities placed on them and whether or not these need revision in the light of wider public or legal concerns. As a dimension of interaction, on the other hand, accountability is located in a range of interactional requirements on the speaker. It is equally layered – it may be there in the overall orientation of the talk (e.g. an account as a response to criticism), as an extended turn (e.g. a narrative or a lengthy explanation) or it may underpin the speaking occasion (e.g. the social worker claiming legitimation through a legal statute). Garfinkel (1967: 22) notes the accountable nature of all talk, as actors are required to justify their actions in a variety of ways to different audiences:

> Any setting organises its activities to make its properties as an organised environment of practical activities detectable, countable, recordable, tell-a-story-aboutable, analysable – in short, accountable.

On some occasions, for example the court or the case conference, professionals explicitly account for their behaviour and justify their assessment and action to others. For example, consider this exchange in which a police officer is cross-examined about the failure to stop rioting (Atkinson and Drew 1979: 137):

Counsel: How many petrol bombs were thrown into it (a newspaper shop)?
Witness: Only a couple. I felt that the window was already broken and that there was part of it burning and this was a re-kindling of the flames.
Counsel: What did you do at that point?
Witness: I was not in a very good position to do anything. We were under gunfire at the time.

The witness produces an account which attempts to downgrade the seriousness of the situation (the building was already alight) and shows that his options to prevent further disorder were severely restricted, as they were under gunfire. This is more than an answer to a question.

On other occasions, accounting is not made explicit. In encounters where the exchange is more conversational (e.g. home visits), accounting practices are more implicit, using devices to resist criticism in order to gain cooperation. For example, Bergmann (1992: 140) describes as 'fishing' where psychiatrists encourage patients to talk about their troubles but play down any criticism in order to gain cooperation.

The production of professional talk and text are inherently accountable occasions. Case files, evidence in court, descriptions to researchers, reports at meetings are occasions on which a social worker justifies their professional and personal identity. As Sarangi and Roberts (1999: 15) note:

> A given professional account will have identifiable linguistic features which are not only durable, but also legitimate and authoritative.

The professional displays competence in using professional words and formulations in their speech and writing to justify their actions and assessments, to counter actual or potential criticism and display authority. In some texts, such accounting is orientated towards the future, displaying to later readers and listeners that action and decisions are correct and in line with rules, procedures, etc. (e.g., Garfinkel on medical reports, 1967: 201; Wilson on judges passing sentences, 1991: 36). On other occasions they are past orientated, and centre on the justification of action in the light of subsequent events already known to the audience (e.g., Atkinson and Drew 1979, on police accounts under cross-examination). In professional talk, there is constant concern with justifying positions in terms of past formulations and anticipated events: speakers continually relate current concerns to previous decisions and set up programmes in terms of future outcomes.

Parents too deploy accounting practices to support their position in interviews, meetings or in court. For example, Silverman (1987: 235) notes how the parents of teenagers with diabetes are caught between allowing them to regulate their insulin dosage themselves and keeping a check on them:

Doctor: How do you thinks she's getting on?
Mother: Very well (.) we only have rows about the tests
Doctor: (.)
Mother: I mean she has to see you, I don't. She's a big girl

Doctor: She's in between. There's a bit of her wanting you to take an interest
Mother: Oh I do. For her own sake. She's growing up fast![1]

The mother manages potential criticism that she is 'nagging' by noting her daughter's age, but then has to defend herself against not 'taking an interest'.

Accounts can be structured in various ways, but generally address the 'gap between action and expectation' (Scott and Lyman 1968: 46). A distinction is made between 'excuses' and 'justifications'. In the former the actor admits that their action was incorrect but was constrained by outside forces. In the latter the actor does not accept the mistakes but pointed to the benefits of their action. Semin and Manstead (1983) also discuss 'apologies', 'requests' and 'disclaimers', each being methods of managing blame and attributing responsibility. However, Potter and Wetherell (1987: 81) note how accounts occur in sequences rather than being located in specific sets of utterances. Over a series of exchanges, actors construct criticisms and defend positions; therefore analysis must consider the encounter as a whole.

Whilst much of this research has been orientated to accounts in ordinary conversation, professional accounting practices are likely to deploy specifically professional as well as everyday formulations. Formulations in professional settings assume institutional significance and can be consequential. As Mehan (1997: 253) puts it:

> It is by invoking the discursive resources provided by these cultural and historical scripts that institutions speak through individuals.

For example, Spencer (2001: 171) notes how the decision by a social worker to deny a service is formulated using 'agency's rules and resources as rhetorical devices':

> Constructing [the social work agency] in this fashion provides a way of accountably making alternative service offers while at the same time not openly challenging the moral claims of service worthiness that are part of this client's self-presentation.

Similarly Mäkitalo (2003) observes how vocational guidance officers account for offers of training or denials of benefits by deploying institutional formulations about the labour market and the efforts of individual job seekers.

As mentioned in the previous chapter, good professional practice requires that 'rational decision-making' activity is displayed – the professional has gathered the facts, considered the options and made a reasonable choice as to the appropriate course of action. However, such activity is interactional and negotiated. Such formulations are not merely constructed as 'rational' but involve the persuasion of particular audiences. Hence, knowledge arising from such occasions is always situated; it requires an account that links the everyday activities and observations with formulations of wider conceptions and concerns of professional practice or government policy. The production of such situated knowledge involves more than the personal reflection of the social worker, as there is a variety of settings in which such knowledge is to be required: the interpersonal encounter (e.g. supervision), the institutionalised event (e.g. case conferences) and supra-institutional scenario (e.g. court hearings), each with different expectations and discursive requirements.

We are suggesting that social workers, their clients and other professionals produce accounts of their actions in everyday interaction. Furthermore, actors are largely unaware of the methods they use to construct and defend their position, what Garfinkel calls 'seen but unnoticed' (Garfinkel 1967: 180). Such research therefore focuses on the detailed study of text and talk which occurred in professional encounters.

Persuasion and power

One particular aspect of accountability is the observation that professional talk and texts are rhetorical in nature because they are concerned with the persuasion of others (Billig 1987), either in face-to-face encounters or when writing for specific audiences. At the same time, social work in particular is constructed on the basis of a concern with factors beyond the immediate talk. The power of the social worker to intervene in people's lives to take action and make statements is itself based on political mandates and legal statutes available outside the encounter (Strong and Dingwall 1983, on mandates). While social workers can take children away from their parents, this power which is clearly outside the face-to-face encounter depends just as much on the local, situated development of a persuasive account (cf. Fairclough 1991 on the distinction between 'power *in* discourse' and 'power *behind* discourse'). Elsewhere we have noted how social workers' talk simultaneously attends to the situation at hand as well as to potential overhearers beyond the immediate encounter, for instance the court (Hall *et al.* 1997b: 201).

There are different takes on the relative power of speakers in conversation. Inevitably, interaction proceeds on the basis that speakers cooperate with one another and abide by certain rules of progression in talk which pushes it forward and enables communication to proceed in the accomplishment of social goals (Grice 1975). For example, if someone asks a question then the other person is expected to provide an answer and whatever they say next will be heard as an answer relevant to a conversational goal or outcome. Such an approach to accounts implies that speakers are concerned with maintaining the normative character of everyday exchange.

In contrast, Billig (1999: 550) examines the limits of approaches to the analysis of language which assume that speakers have equal rights of speakership. He argues that there are occasions in which conversational exchange is more concerned with justification and argument, not seeking resolution or a shared outcome. Speakers aim to persuade, criticise or in some way undermine the other. On such occasions, it is possible that conversational niceties may be circumvented or challenged as a part of the argument. As Bourdieu (1977: 654) notes, speakers want to be believed, even when this happens at the cost of misunderstanding, conversational tensions, etc. Billig (1987: 87) suggests that most conversations have the potential for argumentation once one speaker criticises another's position and the other offers a justification. Questions may be answered with other questions, blaming with counter-blaming. For instance, as we will see in Chapter 5, a failure to take up what the other person says signals the disagreement between a social worker and a client over the necessity and appropriateness of a family therapy service. Thus, what surfaces is a concern with the content of the argument which is not easily categorised into formal conversational methods.

According to Billig, the position taken in an argument may not be explicitly stated but implied:

> Therefore, to understand the meaning of a sentence or whole discourse in an argumentative context, one should not examine merely the words within the discourse or the images in the speakers' mind at the moment of utterance. One should also consider the positions which are criticised or against which a justification is being mounted. Without knowing these counter-positions, the argumentative meaning will be lost.
>
> (1987: 91)

Such an approach to professional talk requires investigating the way in which positions are taken, promoted and defended, both in talk and writing. It draws attention to both the implicit and explicit features of the construction of arguments. This requires a familiarity and insiderness to social work which is usually identified as an ethnographic stance, as much talk may revolve around categories which are not made explicit, but to which argument inevitably attends. As the saying goes: 'there is an elephant in the room'. It is difficult to understand the talk, unless the elephant is made visible.

Blame and responsibility

One salient theme in the literature on accounts is its moral nature. There are two aspects to this: first, there is the moral reputation of the professional and client and, second, there is the professional and client's use of moral formulations. First, accounts in producing justifiable expositions underpin the moral character of the actor. A professional must be able to justify their work, why they have acted in the way they have, what is expected of them in the future, etc. For social work in particular, this has been played out in the media coverage and criticism of child abuse inquiries (see Chapter 9). Douglas (1992: 15) considers that in a society which is driven by concerns of risk management (Beck 1992), blaming systems have developed which treat any unforeseen occurrence as someone's responsibility.

Clients too take up positions in encounters with professionals in which they aim to protect their threatened moral identity. Bergmann (1992) describes how patients manage the 'veiled morality' of psychiatric assessment interviews. Silverman (1987: 249) presents a number of methods used by parents of disabled children to support challenges to their 'moral versions of parenthood'. As we shall see in Chapters 5 and 7, encounters with social workers often require parents to attend to challenges to their moral character.

Second, professional formulations are replete with moral conceptions. Like other professionals, social workers might employ technologies which underpin their decision-making (e.g. research findings, policy statements, psychological profiles, etc.); however what will become apparent in our analyses is the highly moral character of their formulations, descriptions and categorisations. This involves the attribution of blame and responsibility to children, parents, other professionals, and the wider society. Dingwall *et al* (1983: 80) consider:

> Moral character is, then, central to decision-making in child abuse and neglect, as with any other type of deviance. Its ascription, however, is not a straight-forward matter.

Social work is involved with people and their relationships. The social work task is to make judgements and assessments of people's abilities and deficits, in particular regarding the care of their children. Inevitably conclusions will be based on assessments organised around oppositions between (and degrees of) good/bad, responsible/irresponsible, caring/neglecting, dangerous/nurturing, etc. In contrast, people are not normally held morally responsible for illnesses and the technologies of the doctor tend to rely much more on the reading of inscriptions on instruments (e.g. blood pressure, temperature, etc.).[1]

A concern for moral formulations can be seen in both the categories used by speakers but also in the interaction between them. For instance, in the discussion of case conferences (in Chapter 4) we are not just interested in how speakers defend their positions and challenge those of others, but also in how moral formulations are produced in the course of the meeting and how these feed into exchanges between professionals. These instances are interactional in nature, but they are also linked to institutional constructions of people and events which function as accumulative building blocks in the production of knowledge within social work and related institutional settings. Situated social work knowledge has relations to occasions and sites which preceded this one and has consequences for those that follow it.

Parents too deploy moral formulations of blame and responsibility, which are likely to draw on themes of parental privilege and natural love, as a means of reacting to professional challenges. As Slembrouck and Hall (2003) note, these are often sophisticated and carefully constructed. For example, the formulation 'caring but not coping' is a way that parents can admit that they were facing problems but that this should not be used to question their love for their children.

Two important themes follow from this: first, the significance of classification practices and, second, the freedom of and constraints on the speaker. Social workers and clients deploy morally informed categorisations which are not only established and maintained in interaction, but also derive their nature from available discourse routines (e.g. dynamics of complication and resolution in storytelling which shape the formulation of a case). Professional categories may attract moral overtones even when presented as observational facts (for instance, 'poor parenting skills' heard not only in terms of deficiencies in practice, but as an assessment of someone's moral character). Parents are also likely to construct accountability in different ways, drawing on the entitlements of parental authority, with claims to exclusive knowledge about the children. They will also construe professionals in moral terms – e.g. as deceitful or as supportive (Dingwall 1977 on atrocity stories). However they may also incorporate professional concepts: as a mother said in an interview: 'you learn their ways'.

Categories and categorisation

Linked to displays of accountability, a key concept in this book is how professional talk is achieved by the construction and negotiation of and argumentation over categories and categorisation. How do professionals, clients and other commentators deploy categories, sub-categories and their defining attributes to produce competent social work?

Accounts provide the bedrock for categorisation, since it is in accounts (explanations, justifications, attributions of blame and responsibility, mitigations and defensive formulations) that categories are constructed, negotiated and challenged. The ways in which categories are developing in accounts is vividly displayed in a study by Dorothy Smith (1993). 'K is mentally ill: the anatomy of a factual account' is an analysis of a description by a student, Angela, of how she came to recognise that her friend, K, was mentally ill. It shows how the category, mentally ill, is constructed and managed through highlighting aspects of K's strange behaviour. As Smith (1993: 30) says:

> The problem presented by the account is not to find an answer to the question 'what is wrong with K?', but to find that this collection of items is a proper puzzle to the solution 'becoming mentally ill'.

The reader of Angela's account is being persuaded that the attributes and behaviour of K constitute the category 'being mentally ill' (see also Chapter 4).

Also linked to the earlier discussion, we are interested in the moral construction of categories as actors construct and negotiate social work problems, and handle potential blame and criticism. If a social worker contends that a woman is a 'poor parent', then such a claim is likely to require a formulation that demonstrates her as possessing attributes or behaviours which warrant the category of 'poor parenting'. At the same time such a formulation can be challenged by others who might cite instances of 'good parenting'. Negotiation or argument is then required to resolve the dilemma by creating sub-categories, for example as we shall see in Chapter 4, the construction of a 'good mother but a poor parent'.

Theoretical notions of categorisation are widely discussed but are rarely applied to the study of social work. Yet Floersch (2002: 20) notes the crucial role that categories have in establishing a profession's legitimacy:

Problem identification requires the use of subject categories to name and classify the 'it' that practitioners within a social field seek to address. Barbara Nelson points out, for example, how the naming of child abuse as a medical problem was crucial to national agenda setting (Nelson 1984).

Perhaps part of the confusion is that social workers are expected, even required, to name and classify people and their problems in reports, meetings and at court. It is treated as a practical, professional (sometimes scientific) task to produce assessments and recommend action. However as we noted earlier in our comments about evidence-based approaches and social work theory, our approach is to see such processes as complex social, interactional and discursive processes. So when a social worker attempts to define a child or parent, we suggest that it involves more than merely applying social work knowledge to a particular set of family circumstances. Such categorisation processes are inevitably tied up with the contexts within which they occur, the anticipated reactions of various audiences, the discourses available to name and classify, etc. This requires a concern with processes of categorisation in contrast to an approach which sees professional categories as grounded in psychosocial assessment (cf. Little *et al.* 2001).

Categorisation has been considered a central feature of human thought and communication for some time. As a social process, Jenkins (2000) sees it as having individual, interactional and institutional elements. The controversial conclusions of Sapir and Whorf in the 1920s and 1930s that language determines thought fuelled much of the work on language/reality categories. As Whorf (1956: 213–14) comments:

> We dissect nature along the lines laid down by our native languages. The categories and types that we isolate from the world of phenomena we do not find there because they stare every observer in the face; on the contrary, the world is presented in a kaleidoscopic flux of impressions which has to be organised by our minds – and this means largely by the linguistic systems in our minds. We cut nature up, organise it into concepts and ascribe significances as we do largely because we are parties to an agreement to organise it in this way – an agreement that holds throughout our speech community and is codified in the patterns of our language.

Whilst it is inappropriate to summarise debates about linguistic relativity here see for instance Schultz 1990), it is important to outline attempts to theorise the status of categories in everyday action. Categories are spectacles through which we routinely observe and classify the social world. As Lakoff (1987: 5–6) says:

> There is nothing more basic than categorisation to our thought, perception, action and speech. Every time we see something as a kind of thing, for example, a tree, we are categorising. Whenever we reason about kinds of things – chairs,

> nations, illnesses, emotions, any kind of thing at all – we are employing categories.

Research on the use of categories in everyday interaction shows that they are loose formulations, negotiated and reformulated as they are deployed for specific purposes in particular contexts. As Edwards (1997: 224) summarises:

> Verbal categories are resources with which speakers perform discursive actions: they are not just reflections of how they see things or the way things are.

Treated in this way, professional categories, like child abuse, are not obvious from the way in which they are observed, but are the product of constant construction and negotiation.[2] When a child is considered to be at risk, professionals have to manage their versions (evidence, stories, hunches) of what is happening in terms of professional, legal and institutional definitions of child abuse. This is not a matter which takes place inside the social worker's head but one which is carried on throughout various professional encounters – meetings, interviews, court hearings. At the same time other actors – parents, lawyers, journalists – will be carrying out similar categorical construction and negotiation on different occasions and sites. The process and outcome of the construction and the clash of different versions of, for example, whether or not a set of circumstances constitutes child abuse, is the stuff of everyday social work. As we will see in Chapter 8, the categorisation of Victoria Climbié changed on several occasions and was consequential for the actions that followed.

Exploring categorisation in professional talk and texts

There are several concepts that enable a discursive approach to categorisation and accountability in professional encounters – professional categories, argumentation and membership categorisation

Professional and institutional categories

There is much work on how language used in institutions has distinctive characteristics (Sarangi and Slembrouck 1996; Sarangi 1998b). Research has highlighted the way in which such encounters are bounded by attention to rules, mandates, procedures, etc. Goffman's concept of frame has been developed in relation to professional activity (e.g. Strong 1979; Dingwall *et al.* 1983; Tannen and Wallat 1987; Coupland *et al.* 1994). A frame is defined as the way in which actors structure their expectations, how we understand 'what is it that's going on here' (Goffman 1974: 8). For Tannen and Wallat (1987: 206) this means 'what is going on in interaction without which no utterance could be interpreted'. There are rules of conduct or conventions of interpretation which are available prior to an encounter which offer actors suggestions of how to act or how to understand how and why others are acting in certain ways. There is, however, a reflexive aspect to frames (Manning 1986: 255); having deployed the appropriate frame, actors monitor their performance and those of others in terms of that frame. The salience of particular categories can have the effect of framing interaction. On occasion the performance and interpretation of which frame is operating becomes confused (see also Collins and Slembrouck 2004, Sarangi *et al.* 2004). Various examples of this occur in our analysis of the client's experience in Chapter 7 (for instance, the mother describes how what she saw as a normal response to stress during access in a foster home was used to categorise her as a deficient parent).

Institutional arrangements influence (and are influenced by) the establishment of case categories by professionals. For example Dingwall and Murray (1983) note how medical staff on accident departments categorise cases against particular frames. Most of the time a bureaucratic frame is deployed in which patients are conforming and their complaint is routine. Like Strong (1979), they consider that for the most part, patients are assumed to be 'honest, competent and caring' and doctors treated them as rational actors. On occasion, some cases are seen as medically interesting and a clinical frame is deployed, whereas on other occasions patients are seen as deviant and 'special frames' come into play: for example, drunks, drug addicts or children. Dingwall and Murray suggest that such classifications are re-enforced by the social organisation of the hospital – how cases are managed through the system, and once categorised, it is hard to change an established frame. The same is true for social work. For instance, when a social worker begins an assessment, the nature of the referral – e.g. alleged child abuse or financial difficulties – sets a frame around the nature of the ensuing interaction. However, frames are not invoked automatically and there may be conflict as to which frame is appropriate at a particular time. Even so, once established, a category may be hard to change, as has been noted by researchers in child protection (Munro 1996).

Whilst categories are the basis for everyday practice and knowledge of the professional in terms of constructing and justifying their action to various audiences, the nature of the category is often the basis of interaction and argumentation in the professional–client encounter. Mäkitalo (2003) investigates how job applicants and vocational guidance officers negotiate over whether institutional categories, for example an employment subsidy, can be applied to the particular circumstances of the applicant. As Mäkital notes:

> Categories have been generated historically and dialogically in order for institutions to be able to handle or get a grip on the 'social dilemma' that they are responsible for.
>
> (2003: 498)

Mäkitalo (2003) highlights a number of important features of the use of categories in institutions. First, as noted by Dingwall and Murray, categories are embedded in institutional priorities and concerns. Being categorised as one sort of case or another can mean specific routes through the institution, for example whether it is a child protection or a family support case (as we will see in the Climbié case in Chapter 8). Second, whilst categories might appear to be fixed entities, enabling classification against specific criteria, when managed in everyday encounters, they are also dynamic and adaptable, 'when transforming an entity as complex as a person into a case, that is something that the institution can identify and work with' (Mäkitalo and Säljö 2002: 161). Third, establishing categories requires appropriate justification in terms of 'specific traditions of argumentation' (p. 498). This links to notions of accountability discussed above, to define a case as one type or another requires following the proper procedures and forms of explanations. Fourth, there is inevitably an evaluative stance to categorisation in institutional processes. Measuring clients is likely to draw on notions of appropriate behaviour or adequate parenting which involve making judgements in moral terms. As Mäkitalo and Säljö (2002: 162) observe: 'the practice of matching clients to categories is a delicate task'.

Argumentation

It was noted earlier that accountability has rhetorical aspects. Similarly, the construction and establishment of categories involves persuading others and making arguments:

> If the world can be categorised in different ways, then the choice of one particular categorisation can be seen as being part of an argument against another way of viewing things.
>
> (Billig 1985: 97)

The study of categories to locate people and their attributes informs the structure and process of arguments in a professional setting: is this parent caring or neglecting? is this a child protection or family support case? This leads to an analysis of what attributes are constitutive of categories and sub-categories. What range of facts are enough to enable a categorisation to be made and successfully defended? As Gill *et al.* say:

> Rhetorical power does not come merely from the organisation of the claims but from the very categorisations and formulations that are used.
>
> (1991: 20)

Gill *et al.* (1991, unpublished) look at the way that a political speech is constructed to put forward a particular policy and at the same time undermine alternatives. They show that the category 'family' promotes certain connotations and resists others. By deploying attributes about the family and contrasting them with threats, positions are displayed that are hard to challenge. They note the use of certain rhetorical devices to bring off a position; for example, contrasts, three-part lists and depicting assessments as independent of the speaker.

Whilst arguments might take place within conversational encounters, positions may also be worked on beforehand, for example, the defence or prosecution counsel preparing and rehearsing their cases. Overall, as Potter and Reicher (1987: 25–26) note, the study of categorisation can benefit from a study of the 'content of specific categories and the way this is varied in different kinds of accounts'. Billig (1985, 1987) emphasises how negotiation over the attributes of categories can become the sources of argument (1987: 135). Assigning an entity to a category requires a formulation which can be both supported and challenged by particularisation. Can the general category be applied or is this a special case?

> If categorisation refers to the process by which a particular stimulus is placed in a general category, or grouped with other stimuli, then particularisation refers to the process by which a particular stimulus is distinguished from a general category or from other stimuli.
>
> (1985: 82)

Categorisation and particularisation are intimately related since it is only by investigating the interaction between both the general and the particular, that categories and their use can be meaningfully deployed in interaction. This is especially the case when categorisation is studied as a part of developing and defending positions in argument. As we show in detail in Chapter 3 concerning the characterisation of a child sex offender, this is not merely arguing over whether one category is appropriate, but also what constitutes a special case (category plus extra particulars), questioning the boundaries (using particulars to re-define the category) and arguing over arguments (is this way of categorising appropriate?). The manipulation, negotiation and persuasion of categories involves distinguishing similar characteristics but also identifying differences as entities are combined and separated. As Billig (1985: 91) illustrates:

> If one is faced with two stimuli, S1 and S2, where S1 possesses the attributes (a,b,c,d,e) and S2 possesses the attributes (e,f,g,h,i), one can classify the stimuli as being either similar or different depending on whether 'e-ness' is selected as the criterion.

Taking the point further, if e-ness is the defining criterion for a category, not only is there potential for dispute over the amount of 'e' if an entity is to be an example of the category, but also whether the presence or absence of 'a' or 'f' is undermining or confirming the category. For instance, as Dingwall *et al.* (1983) note, social workers can work with clients despite concerns about risks to children; however, when the parents stop cooperating with professionals, the category changes to emphasise the negative aspects. In other words, there is the potential for persuasion and argument about both the necessary attributes of categories but there are also the consequences of identifying subcategories.

Membership categorisation

A number of researchers have developed Sacks's notion of membership categorisation (Cuff 1980; Silverman 1987; Hester and Eglin 1997; Antaki and Widdicombe

1998; Lepper 2000). These devices refer to collections of categories and associated attributes, activities and obligations. For example, when categorising someone as a 'mother' such depictions are linked to other categories in collections (fathers, sons, daughters) and carry with them expectations of appropriate behaviour (loving, caring, comforting). Through member categorisation, speakers and listeners deploy categories and/or attributes of categories, which enable inferences to be made about what is going on.

Sacks (1974) analysed part of a child's story 'The baby cried. The mommy picked it up'. Without stating any relationship, the hearer can infer that mother is the mother of the baby, they are from the same collection, family. This is because 'crying' and 'picking up' are activities and expectations commonly associated with mothers and their babies.

Categorisation analysis develops a complex approach to categories. In contrast to, for example, frame analysis which offers a window on how categories frame complete interactions, these studies show how interaction does not necessarily revolve around a direct examination of whether a category applies. Categories do not necessarily enter interaction in a straightforward and direct formulation. They are often hinted at and negotiated. For example, Watson (1978) studied how in help lines, callers hint at the obligations associated with membership of churches or families. Similarly, categories are constructed through the contrasts with other categories. Smith (1993), in particular, shows how K is established as mentally ill by contrasting her deviant behaviour with the normal behaviour of the storyteller. Hester (1998) investigates how educational psychologists and teachers categorise children as deviant and in need of assessment for special education. The categories are used to locate pupils in terms of, for example, stages of life or maturity, and thereby make contrasts about what counts as normal and deviant behaviour. Hester notes that there are few explicit requests by the teachers for the educational psychologists to act and the categorisations of the problems by teachers are vague. The teachers 'implicate educational psychological intervention' but do not suggest a diagnosis.

Work in this area has investigated the ways in which everyday interaction is concerned with not merely categories but the rights and obligations, activities evoked under the umbrella of a category which is not mentioned (Lepper 2000).

Categorisation at work in professional settings

In drawing together this discussion on accountability and categorisation, some features are outlined which will be explored in the substantive chapters. In terms of the issues discussed so far, we will concentrate our interest on exploring those occasions when social workers, clients and other professionals talk and write about the problems of families involved with social services, that is the categorisation of social work cases.

Whilst the study of categories in talk, associated with membership categorisation analysis, is concerned with how categories might have conversational ends (for example, to produce a blaming – compare Edwards 1991: 517), we are more interested in what we call 'categorisation at work'. How does interaction between social workers, parents and other professionals enable the construction, negotiation and contestation of professional categories themselves (e.g., is this a case of child abuse? is this mother honest or suspect? how do parents resist professional categorisations?). On such occasions, professional categories are both a feature of the interaction but also an anticipated outcome of such processes – professionals are required to produce categorisations of people and events for other arenas and future action. Institutional procedures require that versions of 'what type of case is this' are explicitly accomplished in meetings, telephone calls, case notes, etc. Whilst it is likely that in such processes, conversational strategies, like blaming, persuasion, etc. are also being attended to, wider versions of professional categories are likely to be explicit features of the interaction. At the same time, clients and other professionals may challenge and undermine such conclusions.

Such an investigation necessarily involves moving between interactional and institutional features – professional frames, the content of arguments and the negotiation of categories and their attributes. The work of Mäkitalo, discussed above, is of particular relevance since categorisation in institutions is linked with both the everyday management of professional practices and the context of historically generated institutional procedures, mandates and evaluative processes. In institutional settings, category construction takes place in identified encounters (for example assessment interviews or case conferences) in which categories are well known to (and anticipated by) participants. Hence speakers can be seen as cooperating in producing and refining categories of people and their behaviour. Social workers, clients and other professionals produce detailed descriptions and formulations which feed into emergent professional categories, and form the basis of debate, argument and action. This then requires an interest in 'categorisation at work', that is, the process of negotiating professional categories on occasions specifically organised to categorise people, relationships and situations. It is not suggested that such processes necessarily produce agreement on categories, since both professionals and clients may challenge and undermine one another's formulations, without producing revised versions.

There are particular components which are suggested as integral to such categorisation work – the depiction of events, character and action. Such concepts recall approaches to narrative in literary theory (Chatman 1978, Rimmon-Kenan 1983). Sometimes different features are given greater prominence. For example, Todorov (1977) makes the distinction between 'psychological' and 'a-psychological stories' to show how a narrative can be structured around the plot of the events or the attributes of the characters. Managing the interrelationship between these elements enables the storyteller to approach the storytelling in ways which suit different audiences. Whilst narrative analysis has been an important part of our approach (Hall 1997, Hall *et al.* 1997a), professional encounters and texts are not approached merely to uncover their structural features. A number of the texts are not narratives in the sense of 'fully formed stories' (Labov and Waletzky 1967) but involve complex turn-taking, conflict and interruptions.

Event work

Categorisation of the nature of an event is crucial in social work. How did the bruise on the child occur, was it accidental or non-accidental? In order to make such assessments, professionals and clients are required to debate and contest the attributes of what constitutes accidental or non-accidental. This might involve work on the circumstances of the appointment at the hospital, the doctor's examination of the wound, the plausibility of the explanations, etc. Actors seek to uncover the facticity of the event, using categories like 'seriousness', 'accidents' or 'argument'. Edwards (1994: 218) notes how describing events is concerned with constructing and allocating accountability, leading to blaming, praising or pathologising the behaviour:

> There will be a process of formulating events as routine or exceptional, in that event descriptions can be assembled in ways that claim such a status for a particular event. Events can be given the status of one-off occurrences (items), exemplars (instances) of a script, exceptions to a norm or cast directly in generalised terms.

As Edwards notes, events are described both to identify and categorise them, but also to construct them as routine or exceptional, that is, to locate them within a pattern. This is particularly important for professional assessment. Seeing an event as child abuse depends on identifying it as a one-off or part of a pattern (Hall 1997: 87).

In narrative, events are linked in the plot, imbuing them with significance. Rimmon-Kenan (1983: 15) defines an event as 'a thing that happens':

> One might add that when something happens, the situation usually changes. An event, then, may be said to be a change from one state of affairs to another.

In social work texts where challenges might be anticipated, the change from one state of affairs to another is of particular interest. For example, the re-appearance of a father in the family was seen as changing the categorisation of the case from a cooperative to a non-cooperative family (Hall *et al.* 1997b). How events are depicted and categorised, how they are linked into a pattern and how they produce the plot of a story requires complex creative, rhetorical but also interactional work.

Character work

As with events and plot, the depiction of characters is an important aspect of narrative analysis. The problem with character in the novel is the converse of the character in the professional text. Some literary theories have signalled the death of the character (Barthes, 1975) and reject the notion of the self as an autonomous person. For social workers to depict people as autonomous and categorisable is taken for granted and professionally required. For instance, Parton *et al.* (1997:

109) note how social workers deploy categories of children as normal or otherwise to carry out child protection work:

> All children reported to child protection agencies stand as candidates for possible harm or injury. In order to decide just what sort of a candidate they are, practitioners use category-incumbent behaviours. Breaches of expectable 'child' behaviours are accountable and are of relevance to child protection work.

Similarly, Dingwall *et al.* (1983) consider the importance of assessing the moral character of the parents in order to make decisions about their status as 'child abuser'. They note that in the late 1970s there was a rule of optimism whereby parents were assumed to love their children and therefore ascriptions of parents as 'child abuser' were neutralised. Only when the parents refused to cooperate or the reports of abuse increased did a re-categorisation as child abuser become possible. The categories used to depict someone as a client have a major impact on how the case is handled. Parton *et al.* (1997: 206) describe how a categorisation of a mother as 'alcoholic' appeared in a social work report as justified but remained unexplained. On the other hand in Chapter 3 we will investigate how the categorisation of a 'child sex offender' is explored and particularised in a social worker's description.

Events and character work are used to formulate one another. Dingwall *et al.* (1983: 80) establish the link between depicting events and the assessment of moral character:

> The importance of character has already been hinted at in the way it is used to interpret observed conduct in a prospective-retrospective fashion. This means that past events can be re-analysed to fit the actor's present status, as evidence, for instance, that a parent was 'really' an abuser all along, and to organise the unfolding present as yet further confirmation of the correctness of this ascription.

Parton *et al.* (1997: 103) also note the temporary nature of categorisations, that they are applied and treated as relevant until such time as they are altered or no longer appropriate. To achieve closure as to moral status of parents as caring, abusing, inadequate or dangerous requires detailed and complex work.

Action work

Given that social work descriptions and interactions require the depiction of events and characters, action by professionals and clients follows on as justification and authorisation. Once a categorisation of events and characters is achieved, what is to be done can be heard as obvious. As Toulmin (1958: 97) notes, this may require a 'warrant' to act as a bridge between the facts and the claim. In order to show that the events and characters really did constitute a categorisation, some intermediate statement is required which directs the listener to see the link. In other work we have noted the upgraded nature of such warranting statements, for example 'it really was a very serious matter' (Hall *et al.* 1997a).

Garfinkel (1967: 199) has noted that medical records do not merely relate the facts of the case but justify action. Indeed the facts are often inaccurately recorded since the main purpose of the records is to show to later readers that the procedures were carried out in terms of obligations of professional ethics and the competencies of the agency:

> In our view the contents of clinic folders are assembled with regard for the possibility that the relationship may have to be portrayed as having been in accord with the expectations of sanctionable performances by clinicians and patients.

Similarly, Spencer (1988: 65) notes how information is selected for presentation in court reports in order to justify the recommendation and hence outline the appropriate action:

> According to formal department protocol, the recommendation is a logical and necessary consequence of the facts of the case: the officer's interpretation of the facts lends itself to an appropriate recommendation. Informally, however, a different principle operates. Officers construct and interpret the summary as a warrant for the recommendation which follows: the information contained in the summary renders the recommendation reasonable, rational and in accordance with various bureaucratic protocol.

Garfinkel (1967: 114) notes that such a process works in the opposite direction to a model of rational decision-making – 'the decision-maker's task is to justify a course of action'. The action is decided on and then appropriate information is gathered and displayed in order to support the decision.

Whilst such selection of information and justification of action occurs in retrospect in descriptions or reports, it is likely that in case conferences or professional–client interviews the identification of appropriate action becomes intertwined with events and character work. With particular categories of people and events, then 'what to do' can be depicted as following automatically or even the action justifies the categorisation. Event work, character work and action work are made available to support one another.

Achieving closure

Unlike the categories-in-talk, categorisation work in professional talk has the explicit aim of producing complete, robust versions of particular states of affairs. The aim is closure – what is this person like, how did that injury occur, what should be done now etc. This is the bureaucratic frame which surrounds many of the encounters and texts of professional texts and encounters. Meetings explicitly develop action plans, social workers write reports which assess the facts and professionals and clients have strategies in the talk. How and to what extent they achieve these ambitions is a complex and often contested matter but the aim is to reach assessments, conclusions and decisions.

Such work can be described as rational but, as Cicourel (1976: 49) notes, not in the Weberian version of the idea type, but the everyday properties of reasonable or routine action. Silverman (1987: 38–9) investigates the medical consultation as a 'decision-making' encounter which considers the past treatment history, the preferred disposal, courses of action, examination data, etc. However, the system involves feedback at every stage and as Silverman notes:

> The feedback is a further reminder that the variables should not be viewed as structural determinants of action but as providing a modifiable field of possibilities of action.
>
> (1987: 39)

The institutional frame creates a range of features – reports, expressed opinions, normal procedures, argument – which are available to participants and which are deployed in the encounter to achieve closure. Such closure has much in common with the concept of 'blackboxing' (Latour 1987) developed in the sociology of science: how scientists handle entities as facts which on previous occasions were uncertain and controversial (Gilbert and Mulkay 1984).

It is suggested that construction, negotiation and attempted blackboxing of events, characters and action are central discursive activities in social work texts and encounters. Such activity is seen as achieved through categorisation work and takes cognisance of displaying accountability. Events, characters and action depend on being interactionally accomplished and require categorisation as one type or another.

Summary

We have outlined an approach to the study of professional social work practice which gives a different orientation to concerns with good practice and evidence-based work. We are interested in how social workers, clients and other professionals actively construct, negotiate and monitor their talk and writing in the professional encounters – during policy interviews, in meetings, in case files, during court hearings.

The concepts of accountability and categorisation may be understood by professionals as straightforward and common sense. They need to identify the features of the cases with which they are working and they need to attend to their professional responsibilities. This exploratory review has, however, laid bare the pervasiveness of professional categorisation and accountability as dimensions of all activity. This includes activities which are not normally thought of in terms of establishing categories or accounting for one's actions. The construction of categories is not external to the professional's everyday actions and activities but runs deep in social work talk. Similarly, when a social worker recognises they are responsible for setting up a programme to minimise risk to children, their accountability is also displayed in the very detail of how they perform a set of tasks (and not just in their reporting afterwards). It is thus suggested that a discursive approach to the study of accountability and categorisation is required in which text and talk-in-interaction becomes the focus of detailed study. These concepts are considered to be inevitable features of professional performances, since professional and institutional processes require social workers and clients to construct and defend their versions of what is going on and to do so in ways which appear as justifiable and accountable.

Discourse theory and research provide a number of concepts and debates which support this approach. Research on accountability points towards the study of blame and responsibility in exchanges and the construction and management of excuses and justifications. It suggests a concern with moral and rhetorical features of talk and writing as social workers and clients attempt to support their position and undermine others. Categorisation research points to the way in which actors manage information and opinion by constructing category and sub-categories, with associated attributes, obligations and action. However such categorisation work is complex. It can involve linking instances to wider institutional frames, and constructing events and entities as located in a category but also having particular features. We have suggested that we prefer an approach which is concerned with 'categorisation-at-work', rather than just 'categorisation-in-talk'. That is, we are interested in categories like child abuse or family support which are the explicit topics of debate and negotiation, rather than exploring categories for their relevance in a conversational sequence. We have outlined a number of features which we suggest as particularly relevant to this study – how actors talk and write about events, characters, and actions and how attempts are made to close down debate.

3 Collegial communication in policy review interviews

Introduction

Social workers routinely face a number of situations in which they are required to account for their actions. In supervision sessions with managers, in meetings and at court, their work is subjected to questioning and comment, which might challenge their assessments and inspect their actions. How does the social worker manage such encounters? What strategies do they fall back on for explanation and justification?

The data in this chapter are taken from a series of interviews between social workers who worked for a social services department in an urban authority in the UK and a senior colleague who was carrying out a review of social work policy. This encounter is not a part of everyday work; it is one of several occasions in which social workers are required to justify their actions in professional terms to colleagues (audit, section 8 reviews, etc.). It offers an opportunity to inspect extended forms of social work justification (which are likely to take up considerably more time and engage with more detail than, say, the five minutes allocated to a case summary during supervision sessions). We suggest that the policy review is a site for 'collegial talk' (Atkinson 2004: 13) oriented to the display of competence: 'Competence is at the heart of professional practice, it is legitimation, certification and everyday evaluation.'

The policy review interview constitutes a site where social workers talk about their practice and provides opportunities for explanation, as the interviewees are required to explain and justify their actions. It is also a site charged with potential criticisms which invite rebuttals from the social worker. This particular policy review had been set up to investigate why younger children had been placed in residential children's homes. Such placements were against the policy of the department and were seen as bad practice in social work more generally. It was seen as good practice that, wherever possible, work with families should be carried out with children remaining at home. Where younger children had to enter public care, this should be planned well in advance and the preference was towards foster care. These interviews were used to gather data for the review by investigating the circumstances surrounding instances which were seen as inappropriate decision-making in child placements. The social worker/interviewee was responsible for the case and the policy reviewer/interviewer was from the central planning unit[1]. An explanation of why the placement had been made was invited.

One overarching interest in this chapter is the emergence of a narrative turn in social work accounting practices. The framework of narrative analysis invites attention to particular forms of telling the case which combine what happened to children and their families with an assessment of characters and the constraints and dilemmas of professional practice and managing risk. Of particular interest is how social worker and reviewer manage this process. Although the purpose of this was to justify an inappropriate reception into care, we see that most of the interviews concentrated on 'telling the case', explaining the details and complications of interventions with families, which subsequently resulted in the admission into care. As social work takes place away from the gaze of the public and managers, it is only through telling the case that good work is shown. In Pithouse and Atkinson's (1988: 198) words, 'good work can only be seen through a good account'. Note, however, that 'telling the case' does not necessarily mean that the social workers offer an uninterrupted narrative. In fact, only in one interview was this the case (it is the second set of data in this chapter). More usually, the interview comes with expectations of questions being asked and answers being given and a jointly constructed plot developing across such sequences. At certain points, embedded narratives occur. In an earlier publication (Hall *et al.* 1997b), the contrastive pulls between question and answer and telling the story could be seen as a source of tension: the social worker was initially monosyllabic in her answers to the questions and so managed to negotiate a specific instruction to tell the story in her terms.

A key feature of the explanations is that they trade on the typicality and difficulty of everyday social work. In contrast to the expectations of policy-makers (with recommendations that younger children need never to be placed in residential care) these cases are recounted with an emphasis on the unique details of the case and these are set against the complexities and unpredictability of the social work task. The placement in residential care is hardly mentioned as a problem, even though that was the explicit reason for the interview. Instead, the inevitability of the residential placement is made available as an outcome of dilemmas of everyday work faced by competent social workers who have to balance handling difficult parents, risks to children and a shortage of appropriate resources. By producing an account of professional and competent social work, potential charges of poor child placement decisions can be side-stepped. The importance of 'normal work' as a rhetorical feature to facilitate the smooth running of the organisations has been noted elsewhere ('normal crimes', Sudnow 1965). Similarly, the policy review interview can be seen as a site where the values of the organisation are displayed and attended to by reference to professional ethos and in contrast with the rigidity of policy mandates (Strong and Dingwall 1983).

The policy review interview is thus an intrinsically accountable site, in which the social workers are expected to produce a description of the circumstances of the case in which reluctantly there was no alternative but to place the children in a residential home. As mentioned in the previous chapter, this requires an attention to the way in which case categories become 'particularised' in view of a dispreferred disposal. We would expect, then, categorisation and accountability to be key features of the talk in a policy review interview. Categorisation is central to the policy review interview and to professional work in general. To defend competent social work, both the social worker and policy researcher negotiate the categories which are crucial to social work. They make them visible, grade them or render them relative. In the first interview, child sex abuse is graded: what sort of child sex abuser is this? In the second case, the category of failure to thrive had to be established and made visible: how do we know this is failure to thrive and not, say, a small child? We will contrast these two instances of categorisation.[2] A key feature is the juxtaposition between categorisation (a particular case label, e.g. *'failure to thrive'*) and particularisation (making it individual within the category).

We will also see that social workers need to redefine and re-situate categorisations inherited from other professions within their own talk, making them workable. Social work is frequently required to work to the definitions of others. In the first case analysed here, child sex abuse is a legal category but it also sets perimeters around social work concerns and activities. Similarly, in the second case, 'failure to thrive' is a medical category but with the social implications as a part of the construction process. Such categories have to be broken down into usable observations and formulations which can be recycled for assessment and action. The attributes of the categories (and the instances of behaviour which are seen as supporting them) then become important. For instance, as we discuss in the next section: the father is a child sex offender but there are also other features to his character which particularise the formulation. Social workers can be expected to attach importance to the events, capacities, personality traits, etc. that allow them to deal with the individual case. This does not necessarily undermine the category, but it makes it more malleable and enables it to be appropriated by social work.

Case 1: The 'schedule one' child sex offender[3]

Setting up the interview

The opening of this interview is typical of other interviews in these data. The interviewer's speech is indicated as INT and the social worker's as SW.

Interview 1 – extract 1[4]
01 INT: erm (.) what what were the factors that actually led up to reception into care and ehm and what might have been done had things been available to prevent it now in fact the particular reception into care I had originally thought of was the one in (.) October

02 SW: yes that was only a one night

03 INT: which I realise that [SW: yes] the way I thought we could look at it was the one in use the December one [SW: yes] but the build up through so I perhaps tell me a little bit about your when you took the case on and what was the initial (.) very briefly what were the initial sort of tasks you got involved in

In the opening exchange the interviewer invites a particular method of reporting. The introduction is framed in such a way that a professionally competent social work story is being sought. Rather than challenging the social worker to explain 'bad practice', she is being invited to tell the case in terms which are responsible and justifiable. The interviewer asks both for the reception into care to be located in a set of 'factors which led up to it' suggesting that receptions into care take place in a set of circumstances which require professional explanation. 'What might have been done had things been available to prevent it' offers the social worker an opportunity to point to, say, a lack of appropriate resources to prevent a dispreferred decision. At the outset, the interviewer has provided the social worker with an excuse of both a context and a lack of appropriate provision, undermining a version of individual blame or bad practice. The answer, 'I was inept or made a mistake' is thus unlikely to be available as an option. 'Bad practice' is, then, to be explained in terms of circumstances and resources and not in terms of professional incompetence. Pithouse and Atkinson (1988: 187) observe how failure is usually attributed to others, notably the clients.

In turn 03 of the extract cited above, the sequential nature of events is emphasised since the interviewer talks of the receptions into care as seen through 'the build up'. 'The way I thought we could look at it' offers instruction while highlighting the difficulty which the interviewer anticipates for telling the case: which reception into care do we talk about? where do we locate the storytelling? This could be contrasted with the shared knowledge when a social worker tells a case during supervision (Pithouse and Atkinson 1988: 187). However, unlike the general invitation at the beginning, this invitation here is already more specific, with a more wide-ranging social work explanation expected. The circumstances of the day of the admission to the children's home are not invited as a sufficient explanation. The one-night reception into care in October is downgraded in its significance, as 'only one night' and instead it is formulated as a part of a series of events which culminated in the December reception. That children should enter care for one night is to be explained in terms of a series of family events and social work interventions. In other cases in these data, where reception into care was not part of ongoing social work intervention, explanation was located in the detail of the night of the reception.

Finally, the interviewer encourages the social worker to tell the story in terms of social work developments – 'taking the case on' and being set 'tasks'. These signify an orientation to social work allocation procedures, and a normal way of locating social work explanation in terms of how work is distributed and organised. It is not suggested, for example, that a family history or psychological assessment is appropriate. Even before the social worker has spoken, then, the interviewer has set up the interview as an occasion for talking in terms of social work procedures, professional justification and available resources – all of these are tellable in sequential terms, in the light of relevant background factors. For Pithouse and Atkinson (1988: 194), the case is told as an active 'bricolage', that is:

> bits and pieces of family life are picked out and reassembled into the narrative format of case talk. 'The case', indeed is an occasioned assembly of whatever

fragments of evidence and evaluation the worker weaves together into a plausible story-line.

In addition, we would like to underscore the coordinated interactional nature of case construction.

Identifying the category

Turning now to the first few exchanges we are immediately faced with the categorisation of the father as a child sex offender. This establishes a state of affairs against which the subsequent events, characters and interventions are introduced and is discussed in the context of the efforts of the social workers to protect the children in his family. This case carries in it the potential of turning into a psychological narrative. Events are read off against the categorisation of a child sex offender and this opens up the possibility for character-oriented work, as one of the questions in the background is whether the case is worth therapy and worth keeping the family together.

The social worker responds to the interviewer's invitation as follows:

Interview 1 – extract 2

04 SW: yes I took the case on in October 19— and (.) it was (.) well a high priority child care case because ehm father is ehm a schedule one ehm child sex offender

05 INT: right

06 SW: and we really wanted to make sure that his two little girls were fully protected and (.) so it's been such a solid work both monitoring and trying to improve the family situation to the extent that we could be <u>reeea</u>sonably sure that these two children would be safe in the household growing up (.) ehm initially although we had many doubts we thought there were enough good things going on in the family in terms of particularly of affection and stimulation towards the children that it was worthwhile keeping the family together and put a lot of effort into this ehm

The emphatic use of <u>reeea</u>sonably in 06 already presupposes a situation that the social worker agreed with the father being kept in the family. It anticipates the question in the mind of the interviewer: as the man was a schedule 1 child sex offender, how could you possibly have kept him in the family? The two turns (04–05) set up a contrast which particularises the category: 'yes' this was an extremely serious case requiring solid work, 'but' a more sympathetic view was emerging that it was worthwhile keeping the family together. Such a distinction draws on wide dilemmas in child welfare between aiming to rescue children from dangerous situations and monitoring their progress in struggling families.

In turn 04, we notice that the researcher's invitation to locate the reasons behind the reception into care in terms of social work activity is accepted, with a description of the case as an unambiguous type, a 'schedule one child sex offender'. 'Schedule 1' is a broad category which does not in itself indicate the nature of the incident. Yet, it is a clear categorisation which is extremely powerful in justifying any event, action or character depiction – this case is loaded since it is the type of case which could offer the most extreme of challenges. No details are provided of the nature or instances of the man's child sex abuse. The offences are not described. Nor is there an explanation of the way in which he is a threat to his children, i.e. there is no particularisation of the category itself. The researcher in fact signals, in turn 05, that the category and its seriousness is mutually recognisable. The categorisation is serious enough to both suggest inevitable danger to the children and that every conceivable appropriate intervention should be put in place. Hence, the social work activity is described as 'solid work' and as involving 'a lot of effort' which is based on a balance between 'reasonable safety' and 'enough good things'. The use of upgraded terms about the work done, but with little descriptive detail, here offers an invitation to the interviewer to explore for further questioning the professional task in terms of the nature of the actual work done. Already then we are offered a formulation of a state of affairs based on a mutually recognisable category in which the danger of a child sex offender is translated into the professional formulations of 'work' and 'effort'.

In turn 06, risk management is established as central to the formulation of social work. The principle is developed in terms of being 'reeeasonably sure that these two children would be safe'. The tone used in this phrase is particularly interesting. The first part of the word 'reasonably' is emphasised and extended, but the second part of the word declines in tone and stress. It is not a straightforward emphasis. This formulation highlights a number of crosscutting discursive features. First, the word 'reasonably' plays on different uses of the word. The confidence of the social worker was both 'rational' but at the same time it was 'all that could be expected in the circumstances'. Second, a note of doubt, uncertainty and possibly irony is apparent. The social workers were reasonably sure but not absolutely sure. The 'reeeasonably' contour casts doubt on the whole idea of being sure. This is in contrast to the formulation heard a phrase earlier – wanting 'to make sure that his two little girls were fully protected'. The earlier phrase is the hope, the second the reality. One can never be sure in this work. Does the social worker appear to worry that her 'reasonable' assessment of what was going on is being judged against a too rigid central policy? Either way, the social worker can be heard to instruct the interviewer that their work was motivated by the principle of protecting the children and solid work, but this can never be fully certain.

Continuing with turn 06, risk management is located in a balancing act. The 'many doubts' are balanced against estimates of 'good things going on in the family'. Thus, risk management involves weighing up 'safety' against 'affection and stimulation towards the children'. If these attributes are available in the family, then it appears that the estimates of risk and danger can be reduced. It is the identification and recognition of attributes such as these which determine how the case is formulated. The risks are, by definition, already located in the categorisation of 'schedule one child sex offender' as 'doubts', perhaps not directly identifiable in the everyday behaviour of the family but always present. However, they can be mitigated by the 'good things' and it is on the basis of this that the work commences.

The particularisation of the category 'child sex offender' is now possible and provides the basis of the professional narrative of social work interventions. Note that 'keeping the family together' is a secondary justification after the good things in the family are established. It is not a justification in its own right, because of the dangers of the categorisation of child sex offender. In other cases, keeping the family together is a primary principle of the intervention. Here a lower commitment towards family integrity is suggested.

The initial exchange between the social worker and policy reviewer offers a complex interaction in which a case description, risks and social work ambitions are displayed. This interview was organised to ask the question why these children were admitted into care. However, both interactants appear to accept that this can be answered by discussing the detailed characterisation of the father. The events can be read by understanding the father and his relationship with his family. In this way, both interactants are concerned to understand how a bad placement decision was possible, and both work together to dissipate any blame towards any individual worker. They can be seen to seek to understand and explain the 'bad practice' in terms of the process of ongoing professional work and the management of risk. The interviewer invites the social worker to provide an explanation in sequential themes and professional normal work.

Particularisation and blame

Initially, the categorisation 'child sex offender' unequivocally establishes a state of affairs – the man being a child sex offender means that certain risks are presupposed and interventions must attempt to balance the conceptions of family life and the protection of children. That the category 'child sex offender' is introduced at the outset without details of refinement bears testimony to its all-pervading presence. However, after this categorical opening, the category 'child sex offender' is being particularised in terms of family functioning, with work and effort made available as competent and principled. As the social worker mentions, 'there were good enough things going on in the family in terms of particularly affection and stimulation towards the children that it was worthwhile keeping the family together'. The father was on probation and in treatment with regular visits to the psychiatric registrar and a psychologist. A family therapy programme was set up for the parents and the two children. There was support from a health visitor and a child attendant.

Interview 1 – extract 3

01 INT: what the main concern was was with the father er the father's record and and situation er were there other problems as well in the family that were were worried to you

02 SW: erm parental interaction always seemed to be very odd and we were concerned particularly (clears throat) <u>mother</u> seemed to be a person of many many limitations and most of the parenting was actually done by the father [INT: oh (surprise)] he was carrying out both the practical tasks and the sort of actions

that are (.) <u>emotional</u> bits in a way he was showing he was doing the cuddling . he was erm doing providing the stimulation . the mother was taking a very secondary role

03 INT: (4) and at that stage you w- you you (.) you you were less worried about er (.) I mean what for some the father that there were various allegations of abuse but that really seemed not to (.) er er worry you unduly in terms of that particular development

04 SW: we were worried yes (.) we felt we were walking a tightrope but the balance of probability was that the children were not being being abused (.) as I say because of the level of affection that was going on towards the children

05 INT   and in terms of the family coping (.) were they

06 SW: oh they weren't brilliant at coping ehm often quite chaotic poor hygiene things like this (.) and finances which were always getting into trouble but a lot of the families which we worked with have these sort of problems and they weren't any worse than other families in that respect

In turn 01, the interviewer seems to be suggesting that the family situation and the father's record could be considered separately. He is encouraging the social worker to talk less about the categorisation of the father as a child sex offender and more about what is going on in the family, thereby putting the category aside – at least for the time being. The social worker responds to this by indicating the way in which the mother is failing to parent the children and the father has taken over the tasks: 'practical tasks', 'cuddling', 'providing stimulation'. This is more than the provision of food and clothes. In contrast, the 'mother seemed to be a person of many many limitations', 'taking a secondary role': is it the father who keeps the family together?

In turn 03 we see the reviewer struggling to develop the implications of this complex series of categories. Is the father a risk to the family or not? Note the long pause and the many false starts. Risk management comes to the forefront again (04). There is the social worker's nervous stress on 'emotional' (turn 02) and the interviewer's expression of surprise ('oh'). Arguably the interviewer's turn (03) almost preformulates the social worker's point of view by suggesting the situation may not have called for undue worries. Be that as it may, it is nevertheless attended to as very critical: 'we were worried yes (.) we felt we were walking a tightrope but the balance of probability was that the children were not being being abused'. Risk is played down.

The depiction which follows in turn 06 adds to this assessment: the problems faced by this family are in many ways not atypical. Again it is the researcher who broaches the topic of 'coping'. Up to this point in the interview, the social worker does not seem to be taking the lead. It is the reviewer who has raised the topics of the father's record, the monitoring of allegations of abuse and family coping.

The Canadian episode

Interestingly, while the listener may at this point expect responsibility for getting this family to work to be thrust on the father (he is the problem but he also comes across as the one to work with), this expectation is short-lived, as almost immediately after, the picture is being turned upside-down when the interviewer returns to the topic of the short reception into care in June. Over the next few turns hope is to be invested in the mother's growth (with the help of family therapy offering better chances to protect the children) and a list of negative characterisations is attributed to the father: he is developing an increasing problem with alcohol; there are signs of unpredictable behaviour. We're being presented with a different formulation of the family: the mother and children, without the father. The interview continues with a series of bust-ups, one of which led to the short reception into care in June. A particularly unexpected, dramatic episode now occurs, which, initially at least, seems to support the picture of the mother taking charge of the situation.

Interview 1 – extract 4

01 INT: so this particular at this first reception into care was was very much related to the marital situation [SW: yes yes] and erm (.) at that stage would would any other resources the department had available had prevented that particular reception into care (.) in terms of input into the home or anything

02 SW: (3) no I can't think of any other resources that would have prevented it (.) cos' we were putting in er a [SW: yes] high amount of resources [SW: right] and failed to prevent it

03 INT: right (.) so er (.) that was the the June one (.) right (.) and then

04 SW: I think the crunch point for the family came in August when mother's (.) sister her and sister's husband and his daughter came over from Canada and visited (.) and found (.) I think to their surprise I think (.) and they were just on holiday . they intended to be a holiday but to their surprise that things were really quite bad in this household . the marriage was in a ropey situation . the finances were poor . and the husband was drinking . and the children were being dragged up rather and they were very concerned and actually persuaded mother that she would be better off taking the children out to Canada separated and started a new life in Canada . they were aware that (.) because the children were wards of court there would be legal problems in doing this and they decided to bypass the court system and do it very secretly and no one . the father social services the other agencies knew what was happening until we actually had a phone call from Canada to say they were there which is a remarkable feat

05 INT: that's amazing

06 SW: yes

07 INT: this is also a lot of planning [SW: absolutely] to think it through it shows a good of er organisation

08 SW: organisation (overlapping) on the part of the relatives cos mother couldn't do it on her own

09 INT: good grief

10 SW: so that was the crunch point they left early September er but erm the power of the marriage was so great . that mother found she could not (.) survive in Canada without her husband . and within a day of her arrival she'd started to

contact police and social services crisis care organisations to engineer getting back to this country . and so (.) it was only a matter of weeks before she actually achieved the return

11 INT: right (suppressed, understandingly)

12 SW: and certainly that pushed the marriage into far greater erm difficulties . obviously the husband had been extremely upset that he thought he would never see his family again . and he was very angry . and mother felt when she came back all the father wanted was the children and not her and somehow the marital relationship has never got back on to the same footing . since then it's just gone from bad to worse . so all the crises since then were sort of linked up

13 INT: right (almost inaudibly) so that er they

14 SW: they came back in October

15 INT: right the children came into care over the weekend

16 SW: the end of October yes

17 INT: yes

18 SW: yes

19 INT: what was the circumstances of that

The 'escape' to Canada is a key moment: highly planned, very illegal and yet kind of admirable from a family and parenting perspective. Interestingly, this episode is held back by the social worker: it is a major development which only appears very gradually and it is not introduced or hinted at earlier in the interview. One or two minutes earlier there had been a mention of relatives living abroad and therefore unavailable as a resource to prevent reception into care but the transition to the visit is not an immediate one, as first follows another, more general question about other resources which could have prevented a reception into care. With 'I think the crunch point in the family came in August', the social worker breaks through, as it were, into narrative performance (Hymes 1975). At this point the social worker takes over from the research interviewer, who was about to prompt an introduction to the next episode.

The particular episode is initially told from the viewpoint of the relatives. The description of the family in turn 04 reflect the viewpoint of the visiting relatives. The characteristics are: 'marriage was in a ropey situation', 'finances were poor', 'husband was drinking', 'children were being dragged up'. This is a strongly negative formulation of the family which is in marked contrast to the father as the main carer in extract 3. In as much as the social worker breaks into a narrative of events outside the control of the social worker (the initiative is out of the hands of the social worker), the policy reviewer joins her in appreciating both the narrative and the actions of the mother (turns 05 and 09). Both momentarily sidestep their role, at the same time.

The 'escape' to Canada is a key moment not only in the narrative but also in the interview. In terms of the narrative, intensive work seems to have paid off and weak signs of growth are substituted by heroic action in protection of the children. A final resolution that might have followed from this is that they successfully started a new life in Canada. However, the characterisation turns out not to be definitive and another set of characterisations of the mother and father is introduced: the power of the marriage (turn 10). Families who act this dramatically are very complicated and descriptions of parenting are unlikely to be straightforward. Upon the arrival in Canada, the mother starts engineering a return to Britain: she cannot cope without the father being around. At turn 12 the characterisation reaches the present. The categorisation almost immanent is that of the mother and the father as so consumed with themselves and one another that the children's needs are either increasingly ignored: 'all the crises since then were sort of linked up'. After the Canadian episode, the situation got worse: an angry father; money is kept away from the mother; mother takes the children with her whenever she goes out but feels inadequate to look after them, eventually inviting in the social services to receive the children into care (about a month after their return).

During the telling of the Canadian episode, we can see how the social worker's speech becomes more relaxed. A shared perspective with the research interviewer develops and together they construct an evaluation, expressing surprise and admiration at the mother's unexpected drastic action. So far the mother's 'growth' had been described as one hopeful (but weak) sign (in need of therapeutic support and set off by the father's increasing alcohol problem and unpredictable behaviour). For a while after this stage of the interview, the interviewer's role seems to become more backgrounded. As we can already see in extract 4, he is providing back-channel and asking also what happened next. This stance continues for a while, until gradually the more inquisitive stance (asking for reasons, querying into alternatives) surfaces again. The defining characteristics of the case have been formulated and can now be tested against potentially alternative interventions.

We have seen in this series of exchanges a case told drawing on narrative. Eventually we have identified a plot and a climax. This has been achieved through deploying a number of cross-cutting and not necessarily congruent formulations (the father is a sex offender, but also provides the care in the family; the mother has many limitations but also embarks on a dramatic trip across the world on behalf of the children; the couple cannot be apart but, when together, they are in constant conflict). The contradictions and tensions between these formulations is not resolved, but somehow a narrative is co-constructed. The categorisation in this context is complex and 'unfinalised', meaning that the social worker finds it difficult to impose definitive descriptions of the people they work with (cf. Bakhtin 1984). This narrative appears to be assembled as it was told in response to the interviewer probing, rather than clearly worked up beforehand (as in the case we analyse next).

Case 2: Failure to thrive

In contrast to the categorisation of 'child sex offender', the case of 'failure to thrive' is established accumulatively. It appears in a long, uninterrupted narrative, detailing interventions and interactive contact with the family and various agencies. A detailed narrative analysis of these data appeared in Hall *et al.* (1997a). We will summarise this analysis and concentrate on the ways in which the categorisation of the case was achieved. Whereas in the first case the categorisation was introduced at the beginning of the interview and the characterisation of the parents was made clear, here the category of 'failure to thrive' is made available as the events of the story unfold, the states of affairs are built up, the characters gradually appearing through their actions. The second set of data are also different from a narrative perspective. It includes a clearly bounded narrative, with speaking and listening roles established at the outset.

The social worker's first utterance establishes a frame for the storytelling. The social worker silences the researcher by claiming the floor in a direct and strong rhetorical bid for an extended monological turn (cf. story-prefaces, Sacks 1967 in Coulthard 1977: 82ff.).

Interview 2 – extract I

```
01 SW:  well look I'll speak to because I can I can
02 INT:  I'll leave it to you (laughs)
```

In this way the social worker offers a clear instruction to the researcher that this will be an 'I' story, told from the point of view of the social worker as a 'hero'. It means that not only is the social worker making a claim to tell the case in his terms without guidance or interruption but that there is an overall logic to his account which any interruption might challenge. For the first 12 minutes of the interview, the reviewer is reduced to backchannel, as the case is being established in the social worker's narrative.

The problem for the storyteller is that the diagnosis of 'failure to thrive' is potentially open to other interpretations. Medical research in the field often constructs the category without making requirements about the links to parental blame or child neglect. Social work writers, on the other hand, are more likely to deploy the category by adding riders about neglect and abuse. For example, Gilmore (1988: 52) make an inevitable link:

> There can of course be an almost endless range of mixed causes whereby a medical condition may indeed be responsible for a child's failure to thrive, but that such a condition occurred or was not dealt with sooner, or did not have a persistence in treatment, may be partly or wholly due to the neglect on the part of the parents.

However, such a link has to be established, as child neglect is not presupposed by the use of the category. The requirement to particularise 'failure to thrive' with adequate social information added to the medical information is, then, critical to the construction and visualisation of the category of this case.

Labov provides a way of analysing the structure of narratives in terms of evaluative problem-solving activity using the 'episodes' of orientation, complication, evaluation and resolution (Labov and Waletzky 1967; Labov 1972). Following his model for the analysis of narrative structure, four phases can be detected: the initial discovery and the social worker's initial successful activity (orientation), the social worker's eventual failure (complication) and finally the confirmation of blame (evaluation) and removal of the children (resolution). The four phases, it is suggested, create a justification for the most extreme use of the police powers available to the social worker: to remove children from their homes against their parents' wishes. At the same time, the apparent ease with which the social worker delivers the narrative is significant and suggests that a similar presentation has been performed in other settings (for instance, the court). The apparent straight-forwardness with which the narrative here can be mapped on a linear structure itself begs a number of questions about narrative performance in social work accounting, especially when it is contrasted with the way in which in the first set of data the narrative is constructed in response to interviewer probing. We will address these questions in the concluding section.

The narrative structure of an account of failure to thrive

At the outset, the social worker provides a narrative orientation – an initial description of the characters and a first set of events to which the listener is invited to orient. He starts with being allocated the case, as the child was in hospital as a result of medical concerns that he is underweight. There is no description of the parents, no mention of their names nor prior history, the only characteristics being their young age and housing situation. However, the seriousness of the case is made available through the extreme concerns of the medical staff: there is the voice of the GP 'who was *very* concerned', the hospital felt 'it was a clear case of failure to thrive'. Although no clear link is made with parental neglect, the mother's lack of cooperation with the hospital staff resulted in a court order requiring the child to be kept in hospital. Thus, a categorisation has been made available and located within the circumstances and characteristics of the family. It is still without the details which are required for categorisation and particularisation which will lead to a moral assessment and blame. At this point, there is a case to answer and it is this task which opens the way for the social worker's intervention.

The orientation continues when a series of interventions are narrated which initially appear to be successful. The introduction of this social worker appeared to reap instant rewards, for although there were problems of placement and contact, the 'assessment went very well'. The social worker developed a 'relationship with the mother' and was able to handle the case sufficiently well to recommend a supervision order at court – a lower tariff disposal. The mother is portrayed as hostile but there is enough cooperation for social work to be possible.

Next, the social worker describes a series of failed interventions and shows frustration at the new situation. The change in the state of affairs is indicated as an abrupt reversal of the parent–social worker working relationship ('as soon as the baby went home very sadly the parents refused to cooperate'). Affective phrases illuminate the social worker's disappointment at this change ('very sadly', 'unfortunately'). Interventions which had been set up in the assessment phase are now seen to collapse. In terms of narrative structure, this represents a complication. Throughout this stage the social worker is at pains to describe his reasonableness and his attempts to engage with the parents. The voice of the parents is still not available nor is there any suggestion as to why their position has changed. Furthermore, whilst failure to thrive is located in the family with concerns about a new baby, the parents are still not blamed directly for the condition – the condition is still portrayed as medical rather than child neglect.

The baby is admitted to hospital and diagnosed as having reflux. The medical intervention now offers the opportunity for blaming the condition on the parent's handling of the children. Although the mother was instructed how to feed the baby, the baby failed to put on weight at home but she did put weight on in hospital when fed properly 'so the medics felt that clearly it was a question of the way the baby was being handled and fed'. The contrast between the hospital and home is now proven and failure to thrive is established in terms of the parents' inability to look after their children. Decisions are made and decisive action is outlined. The social worker still tries to get the cooperation of the mother but, without this, he is forced to resort to a drastic intervention, i.e. remove the children against the wishes of the family with a court order. By describing the court order and the admission into care, the narrative receives a resolution which resolves the complication. A coda follows: 'that in summary is the case'.

Categorisation and blame

In this narrative, the specificity and implications of the initial categorisation of failure to thrive are delayed. There is no clear link between the condition of failure to thrive and the characterisation that this was the result of parental neglect. The initial character depiction outlined some features which could have formed the basis of an unsuitable mother – young, homeless with a delinquent partner. However this could not in itself be used to create a depraved characterisation, nor is it being developed further.

Interview 2 – extract 2

SW: on being taken there erm the hospital felt that this was a <u>clear</u> picture of a failure to thrive the child was . as I recall off the top of my head . I think it was two and a half kilos under weight was very dehydrated and in fact had the situation been left for longer the child could have died [INT: mm] the child was admitted and what then happened was that erm the mother erm (.) the staff found the mother very very difficult very hostile uncooperative erm and the the situation er caused so much anxiety that a place of safety was taken and the child was kept in the hospital [INT: mm]

This particular extract establishes the medical condition of failure to thrive and an uncooperative parent, both using upgraded terms. A causal link between two may be implied but it is not made explicit.

In a similar vein, in the next extract, a characterisation of 'poor parenting skills' is implied by the mention of services offered, but with no explicit description of the parents' deficits and how it might contribute to the category of failure to thrive.

Interview 2 – extract 3

SW: we then had a double problem that (.) workwise we were putting in the family welfare association who were meant to be there to <u>counsel</u> the family and to offer them erm primary care which would involve them developing their parenting skills [INT: mm] so they were heavily involved

So, it was the efforts of the hero and his colleagues which was the main way in which the case was developed and the unfortunate state of affairs was displayed. Blame, then, appears to be based on contrasting the responsible character of the professional with the uncooperative parents. However there is still no character depiction of a 'bad' mother or father, just a 'bad' client.

A more explicit link between failure to thrive and parental neglect emerges in the resolution of the narrative.

Interview 2 – extract 4

SW: the baby while (.) in hospital had actually put on weight [INT: yeah] having been fed under a normal regime indicating so the medics felt that clearly it was a question of the way the baby was being handled and fed (.) [INT: mm] what the mother came to that case conference but went off in a temper before we could explain the recommendations or the decisions

When the blame finally does appear, it is based on a particular logic rather than a description or a particular set of observations. The parents have failed because the scales proved that, unlike the nurses in the hospital, they were unable to provide a feeding regime that enabled the child to gain weight. There was still no description of the parents' lack of knowledge or love for their children, but instead an assumption that parents who do not feed their children have failed and in such circumstances the children must be removed. No intentionality is attributed to this act, however: the parents' refusal to cooperate can be heard as parents who are not acting to promote their children's well-being.

In contrast to the establishment of the category of 'child sex offender' in the first case we analysed, we have seen in this section how, gradually and through a narrative, 'failure to thrive' is made available as a 'clear' category. Even though medical definitions were available at the beginning, a social definition and its associated blaming is made available through the display of events and states of affairs. This process of gradually establishing the events which led to the proof of failure to thrive means that the category is made available through its particulars. However, the characters of the parents, their attributes as a mother and father and their points of view remain ill-defined. They have been portrayed as violent and uncooperative clients, but this is not seen as either necessary or sufficient to establish the case as 'failure to thrive'. Perhaps this is a response to the difficulty of translating the medical category of 'failure to thrive' into social categories which require blame and responsibility.

Telling a case

Both categorisations and narrative structure can be recognised in these interviews as central to the way in which a social work account is tied together. In the first case, a category is established at the outset. While the question/answer phase harbours an underlying narrative in that it is organised around events, it is only with the Canada episode that a more monological form becomes available which takes the interviewer up to the current state of affairs. The significance of the immediate categorisation in the first utterance is made available as events unfold but after a 'crunch' episode the narrative structure is completed. The categorisation has however become complex: underscoring the category of 'child sex offender' while establishing child neglect in the capacities of and relationship between both parents. In the second set of data, an explicit narrative structure is established at the outset, and a categorisation is introduced in a limited (medical) formulation. The category as a matter of child neglect is delayed, only appearing in the resolution of the narrative.

Pithouse and Atkinson (1988: 184) argue that all social worker accounts are structured around narratives:

> Typically they [case talk] are ordered around coherent narratives. The case is shaped and ordered through the account. The narrative itself conveys, often implicitly, the worker's evaluative stance towards the work which is recounted.

Our contention is that it is the juxtaposition of narrative with categorisation which brings off the account. An account would not work without a categorisation and a categorisation invites a narrative turn in the talk. Neither the category of 'child sex offender' nor the category of 'failure to thrive' can itself justify the reception into care. The categories have to be shown to lead on to child neglect or abuse.

In the first data set, the particularisation of the category of 'child sex offender' invites character work. Rather than concentrating on the definitive features of the initial category, risk is located in the complexities of the characters of both mother and father and their volatile relationship. Events are seen as a direct consequence of the 'sort of persons they are' and 'the kind of relationship they have'. In the second data set, event work pushes the narrative forward, with scarce explicit descriptions of character and an absence of attributes other than what can be inferred from the parents' actions. This feeds into wider debate about event versus character-oriented narratives (cf. Chatman 1978).

One would assume that social workers will have a preference for character-oriented narratives. Yet, their work will tend to be organised around events which spark off intervention. Because their involvement with clients will tend to be long-term, narratives will rarely be finalised. It may be expected though that different audiences invite different narratives. Social workers' accounting practices will revolve around explaining events in terms of character as well as showing character through events. Events will never be enough in their own right if they do not lead to characterisation. Similarly, a characterisation is itself not enough as it has to be operationalised through events and can be undermined by subsequent events. The 'bricolage' which Pithouse and Atkinson (1988: 194) identify in case talk is not arbitrary, but has to be grounded in the credibility demands of various audiences.

Ochs and Capps (2001) discuss the relationship between the narrative and the conversational in terms of unfolding frameworks for understanding events. Some narratives will be launched without necessarily knowing exactly where they lead. Others will come with a sense of unity through foreshadowing and an expectation of finalisability. The first interview differs in this respect from the second interview. In as much as 'wait I'll speak' in the second interview counts as a signal to the reviewer that the only way he will understand the decision is if he sits through the whole story and the point of the story is to confirm the element of risk warranted by the first mention of the category of 'failure to thrive', the first interview does not end with a corroboration of the initial category in subsequent events. Quite the contrary, the initial category of 'child sex offender' is much less central to the establishment of the parents being blamed for being so consumed with themselves and one another that the children's needs are ignored. As one reaches the end of the interview, one may indeed have almost forgotten about the early categorisation of the father. In short, to the extent that a narrative turn is almost inevitable in the context of a policy review interview, such cannot be concluded to predict that a narrative will take the form of an extended monologic stage or that an early categorisation will foreshadow narrative unity of the kind where at the end of the narrative, the teller has sought to demonstrate the point s/he set out to make.

If it is accepted that this review was based on an assumption that admitting young children into residential care was bad practice, the problem for the social worker is to demonstrate to the reviewer that s/he acted professionally, was competent in the assessment of the case and attempted interventions (but despite all, the admission occurred). Therefore, as Pithouse and Atkinson (1988: 198) stress, the rhetorical skills deployed by the professional worker in telling the case become constitutive of the worker's expertise. Complexity is inevitable.

Conclusion

This chapter has attempted to apply our theoretical framework of categorisation and accountability to two policy research interviews. We have seen how in two contrasting cases categories and their attributes are made available to blame clients and deflect from any criticism of social workers' own practice. Using characters, events and states of affairs, two contrasting social work categories have been used to establish these cases as the site for competent professional work.

In neither case were the 'inappropriate', 'bad practice' child placement decisions addressed directly. Rather, the formulations were set in a context of competent work and the construction of complex professional categories. If you understand the professional context you would not question the child placement decision. There is almost an arrogance about the formulation – how can you question my decision without understanding the professional context? Only when you have travelled with me through the events, states of affairs and met the characters can you begin to understand the circumstances in which the child placement decision was made. It is thus a process of 'translation' (Callon 1986), taking the listener through the sites of social work practices as the 'obligatory rite of passage' (Latour 1987) to talk about social work, social work decisions and social categories.

When professionals talk about their clients, we see that they are acutely aware of the complexities which accompany their work. In both instances, the storyteller has responded to the requirement to justify a reception into care with long narratives which include unresolved categorisations and interlocking events. In both instances, the account has been framed within an all-encompassing narrative. This has enabled them to display their outline of the case and draw in the listener. The talk is collegial, and, as mentioned at the beginning, the display of competence is central to it. Our analysis puts in perspective again, the problem of what constitutes evidence in professional practice. As Atkinson (2004: 22) notes:

> Contemporary emphases on evidence-based medicine too frequently treat 'evidence' from purely normative and decontextualised standpoints. There is pressing need for analyses of how the different varieties of practical evidence is constructed, conveyed and evaluated through studies of medical talk in naturally-occurring settings. These analytic interests are not confined to the examination of collegial work in medical settings. Evidence and competence are implicitly commented upon and evaluated in the course of professional talk in a variety of occupational and bureaucratic settings.

4 Inter-professional decision-making in a case conference

Introduction

Much of the everyday work of social workers in the UK is orientated towards meetings – planning and organising them, producing documents, managing the discussion and carrying out tasks set by the meeting – so much so that the mandate for social work is frequently located in such meetings. There are several types of meeting in social work with different formal or organisational requirements.[1] Reviews of the progress of children in public care are the subject of statutory regulations, as are child protection conferences. Other meetings are less formal, for example, allocation meetings, strategy meetings or family group conferences, where concerns are discussed and services reviewed.

This chapter investigates talk in a child protection conference. The organisation and function of child protection conferences are set out in official procedure, including a requirement to construct and ratify a categorisation, i.e. is there sufficient concern about this family for the child's name to be placed on the child protection register and a child protection plan to be set out?[2] Participants at child protection meetings include a range of professionals – social workers, teachers, health workers, police, residential and day care staff – and it is seen as a key site for agency collaboration to ensure that interventions with families are coordinated, an issue which has frequently drawn government and media criticism (Reder *et al.* 1993; Laming 2003). Parents and children are usually invited to attend such meetings, although the extent of their participation varies (Thoburn *et al.* 1995; Hall and Slembrouck 2001). The explicit purpose of meetings is to make decisions and plan services, but to do so in line with departmental procedures and requirements, so that they tend to be chaired by managers or independent reviewing officers. It has been noted that unlike, for example doctors, social workers attempt to share the risks and responsibilities and promote their role as acting on behalf of the meeting (Hallet and Stevenson 1980).

As social work meetings have a variety of functions, they are likely to have competing priorities, yet achieving consensus is vital. Boden (1995: 86) notes the 'synchronicity' of decision-making in organisational meetings. Adelsward and Nilholm (2000) also note the orientation to consensus in meetings between parents and teachers. Not surprisingly social workers and their managers are concerned about the process, constitution and outcome of meetings. They are likely to be discussed in advance, invitations to attend are monitored and appropriate timing considered, particularly on the part of the chair of the conference (Farmer and Owen 1995: 84). In short, they are surrounded by strategic activity or, as Corby *et al.* (1996: 488) say, they are 'stage managed'. Consequently, it is not surprising that other professionals (Simpson *et al.* 1994: 224) and clients (Corby *et al.* 1996: 480) often see such meetings as tightly controlled and the decisions made in advance. A number of commentators have noted the lack of disagreement in meetings and see this as the professionals constrained to present a united front to parents (Bell 1999: 448; Corby *et al.* 1996: 488; Farmer and Owen 1995: 86).

Another complication about child protection meetings is that although formally the function is to consider whether to place a child's name on the register, at the same time other actions may be carried out by professionals but not overseen by the meeting. For example social services may take the child into care, education may start a special needs assessment or the police may instigate a prosecution. Such serious actions are likely to be discussed at the child protection conference but the meeting does not have the remit to ratify such action. The ambitions of the meeting may be constrained by such outside pressures as, for example, access to resources or the decisions of senior managers, other agencies or courts.

Given their centrality to social work practice, it is surprising that there are few studies of what goes on in social work meetings. Research has tended to rely on interviews with participants (Bell 1996; Farmer and Owen 1995; Corby *et al.* 1996) or the researchers' assessment of meetings (Thoburn *et al.* 1995). Research on other meetings has noted their importance to the ongoing performance of organisations (Boden 1995: 99). Adelsward and Nilholm (2000) note how meetings are used as a resource to structure ongoing parent–teacher interaction. In this analysis, we concentrate on one meeting, a child protection review, and how certain forms of evaluative talk and strategic action appear in such contexts.

Constructing client character

This chapter develops the concepts of character construction and its relationship to categorisation by considering how the client is depicted and assessed in a social work meeting. Characterisation is about 'what sort of person are we dealing with?' Categorisation is about 'what sort of case is this?' We are interested in how the two come to affect one another. In everyday interaction, descriptions of people are strategic and contextual. On occasion, speakers may wish to provide a definitive portrayal, but also depictions are often pitched with a hedged commitment or uncertainty. As we saw in Chapter 3, a characterisation can be effected by a narrative being told. In case conferences, on the other hand, characterisation is more likely to be oriented to the immediate purposes of the meeting and it will tend to develop across the various contributions. Professionals in particular monitor their performance in meetings. As a result, descriptions are likely to anticipate audience reaction and the task at hand.

Case conferences offer a particularly interesting site since character construction is open to immediate debate and challenge, but this happens in an arena aimed at cooperation and consensus. There is a requirement to reach agreement about whether the child should be placed on the child protection register, if necessary by 'a show of hands'. In this analysis, we suggest that such agreement involves reaching consensus about the moral character of the client, in this case the mother. Once the mother can be successfully depicted and categorised, the conference can come to a decision about whether to register the child.

For the professional, how they perform at the conference has implications for their competence and standing. If a professional can produce the most telling character description or most accurate assessment which gains the support of others, then both their personal esteem and the standing of their agency can be enhanced amongst fellow professionals.[3] The client too is likely to be aware of the need to monitor their performance in case conferences and to display cooperation with the professionals (Dingwall *et al.* 1983: 92).

To summarise, the notions of character depiction, contested categories and audience can help our understanding of the nature of talk and interaction in social work meetings. It is hoped that this analysis will also shed light on the professional concerns outlined – how performances are monitored, how others are persuaded, how consensus is managed with parents and professionals and whether this can be considered 'groupthink'? Our analysis will explore how far the construction and negotiation of the character of the mother is managed in the discussion and decision-making of the meeting.

Introducing the case conference

The meeting we analyse is a child protection review, taking place in a social services office in a large city in the UK in the mid-1990s. The conference concerns a family consisting of a mother, Kathy, and her three children, Ellen (aged 12), Neil (aged 5) and Terry (aged 3), and has been arranged to review an earlier decision to place the children's names on the child protection register. There has been ongoing contact with the family for many years and recently Neil was taken to hospital with an injury. All the children were placed on the child protection register, because of this incident and ongoing concerns of 'neglect' of the children.

The child protection review is arranged by the social worker and chaired by a senior social services manager. Those present are teachers, day care staff, a health visitor, education welfare, a family therapist, the police, a foster parent, and a council solicitor. Kathy, the mother, is also present but not the children. Permission to tape record the meeting was obtained from all participants. The meeting is structured around each professional's verbal report on the service they are providing and how they assess the current risks to the children. The social worker responsible for managing the 'protection plan' is the first speaker and provides an overview of the services and concerns. The chair asks questions of each professional to expand on key points but in general professionals do not speak outside their turn. The mother is able to comment and ask questions at the end of each professional contribution although on occasion she interrupts other speakers or engages in a dialogue over particular issues. After all the professionals have made their contribution, there is a general discussion of the key points and the chair summarises the current concerns and future plans. The decision to keep or remove the children's names from the child protection register is made at the end of the meeting by the key organisations – social services, education, health and police. Whilst the child protection conference is mandated to make decisions about registration, it is likely that any aspect of professional involvement with the family is discussed, and linked to the 'protection plan'.

Our argument is that in the case conference, professionals seek cooperation with one another in character work. In this case, the moral character of the mother is established in order to assess her love and care but also her deficiencies and the risks to her children. The nature of description and evaluation in the meeting is organised around depicting the mother's character rather than focusing on the nature of abuse the children have faced. When the meeting has successfully categorised the mother, they are in a position to bring about a shared decision. It is not suggested that this is the explicit aim of the chair, but that other participants intervene to make their contributions in ways which can be heard as adding to the character depiction of the mother. Even if there is 'disagreement', it is discursively approached as refinement.

In our analysis we will demonstrate how the construction of moral character is achieved through three different but overlapping rhetorical and interactional features.

Contrastive character work

Parton *et al.* (1997) note how the moral character of a mother is constructed through comparison between normal and abnormal behaviour. Sometimes there is direct comparison where abnormal behaviour is contrasted with what is characterised as normal behaviour. Smith (1993: 26) develops the notion of contrast structures, where a person is depicted as mentally ill by directly contrasting the subject's abnormal behaviour with what normal people were doing:

> We would go to the beach or the pool on a hot day and I would sort of dip in or just lie in the sun, while K insisted that she had to swim 30 lengths.

Hall (1997: 61) notes how deviance is established in social work talk by inferring rather than stating the contrasting normal behaviour: 'for instance X who is aged 7 has moved 30 times in his lifetime (-)'. It is sufficient to outline only the abnormal behaviour since it is assumed that the listener will 'hear' the contrast – that children aged 7 will not normally move so often. Contrasts are suggested as a key feature where the aim is to establish a deviant or discredited character.

Consensual character work

The consensual nature of case conferences has already been noted. By jointly constructing the character of the mother, each professional contributes to the shared task at hand. There are three aspects to this. First, claims about the character of the mother are made by explicitly recruiting the voices of colleagues and other agencies to support their claims, for instance 'A.N. Other agrees with me on this.' Second, participants are specifically invited to endorse aspects of the character work which is taking place, for instance 'X, do you agree with what Y just said?' Such work both recruits support for the speakers' claim and sets the agenda for other contributors. Third, the collective nature of assessments and opinions are expressed at key stages in the discussion as summary points (usually by the chair), in order to emphasise that agreement is achieved and suggesting a categorisation 'if we agree that X remains the main problem, then . . .'. Once achieved, such a categorisation becomes a platform, a 'black box' (Latour 1987), on which other agreements can be sought, but it also becomes harder for others to challenge.

Cumulative character work

Developing out of consensual character work, we see that characterisations are built on top of one another, for instance 'we found that but also we found . . .'. Taking up the invitations to agree, speakers are able to build on the accumulating characterisation of the parent, appropriate it and make it theirs. Here agreement becomes less straightforward as the adding on of claims and experiences might be heard to alter the depiction of the mother and its consequences. This is a key aspect of categorisation work more generally, as properties of categories are negotiated and established. Sacks's work (1992) on membership categorisations notes the way in which more complex versions of characters are developed by negotiating the incumbent properties which hint at a category (rather than making the category explicit; cf. Atkinson and Drew's (1979) observation that the naming of a place may identify a religious type). Although there may be no explicit disagreement or dismantling of other claims, subtly different positions can be put forward in a meeting. Examining school meetings with parents of children with disabilities, Adelsward and Nilholm (2000) note how a mother may subtly re-negotiate the identity of her daughter in more positive ways without incurring explicit disagreement.

These three features overlap and are intertwined in the joint moral character of the mother. They form a key part of the interaction in the case conference and have been noted as central to talk in other meetings, as Boden (1995: 90) says:

> This contrastive yet cumulative subtext of persuasion is what negotiation is all about. It is built into the sequential structure of talk as action.

We now examine extracts from the meeting in terms of these features of character work.

Good mother/poor parent

At the beginning of the meeting, the social worker has been invited to lay out the main features of the case. Her outline is interrupted by the mother's [KM] late arrival. After introductions, the chair [CH] invites the social worker, Annie [SW] to continue:

Extract I

43 CH: where were we so I think we've back just about can you carry on

44 SW: yes I think ehm it is to do with ehm exercising adequate control really and putting down firm boundaries for all of the children and ehm and . although we've been through some very difficult times with Ellen ehm (.) but I can see now certainly Kathy . when I spoke to you last week . was talking ehm quite specifically about difficulties now arising with Neil (.) ehm along similar lines to things about being able to ehm to parent him . and and to be firm and consistent with him . so he gets clear messages about what's actually expected of him ehm (.) and I think my concern is really for the future I I'm concerned that if things don't change for the children . if things aren't clearer for them about what what's expected of them . and how they should act . then I can see that as they get older . it's going to become increasingly difficult for Katherine to actually ehm to continue to control them

45 CH: ok (2) can I just check on ehm (.) and I'll come back to you Katherine in a second to check the whole thing out . can I check on on . are there aspects of parenting . I just wrote down if you like the nurturing and emotional aspects of the relationship between say Katherine and either all the children or individual children (.) can you comment on that

46 SW: yes I (.) my feeling is there's a good relationship in terms of – I don't question at all Katherine's er love for her children or their's for her . I ehm I think they're very clearly very very attached and very fond of her ehm (.) I suppose I can see though that that that can be jeopardised by other things . going back again to er controlling them ehm (2) but in terms of relationships . the actual basic relationship . I think that that love and affection is there

47 CH: ok ehm another bit of parenting just occurs to me . there might be others . if people check them out . but in terms catering to their physical needs for instance food clothing warmth

48 SW: yes . well I think at the last conference we certainly we talked about food . and I think that that's been an area of concern ehm

49 KM: but I've sorted all that out now

50 CH: can you (.) I'll come back to you (.) go on Annie you say you say your bit and then we'll

51 SW: we we did actually ehm try to involve er a home economist right (.) in a few minutes I can put I can read out her input ehm (.) my concern is that when I do visit I do see the children eating a lot of sweets ehm and other things crisps and I'm very conscious of that . now obviously when I visit that's just a snippet of the day ehm . but I do observe that (.) ehm maybe other people can comment

from what they've observed about diet . and I know that there have been some
concerns about Ellen and her weight gain (6)
(SW goes on to talk about clothing)

The chair offers the social worker the opportunity to describe the key features of
the case, drawing on the plans from the last meeting, listing what was decided and
what has happened since. The social worker is then given the opportunity to
develop her position further by engaging in an evaluation of the mother's parenting.
This is developed in terms of character work, that is, Kathy's parenting abilities are
explored in terms of an evaluation of her character – being inconsistent, unable to
control or feed her children appropriately. The social worker uses the 'I' voice to
justify her evaluation and in particular she draws on what she has observed.

Let us begin with the contrastive work being undertaken here. We see two types
of contrast at work: contrast with an external entity (good parenting as it exists
elsewhere) and contrast internally (Kathy as a good mother but an inadequate
parent). Kathy's character is built up through contrasts with normal behaviour, in
this case through setting out certain standards of good parenting and noting how
Kathy falls short. The social worker lists a series of concerns about Kathy's parenting
– exercising adequate control and boundaries, being firm and consistent, the
children's diet, concerns about weight. Each of these concerns is posed as problematic and as constituting deficient parenting. For example, in turn 44 the concern
is about 'exercising adequate control'. Indeed, 'be able to ehm parent him' is seen
as constituting being 'firm and consistent' and giving 'a clear message about what
is expected'. The consequences of such deficient parental control are also laid
out: if the children are not made clear about what is expected of them, then
they will become out of Kathy's control. The link between 'lack of control' leading
to 'out of control' is established, so the children's bad behaviour is portrayed
as directly caused by Kathy's deficiencies. Any sign of the former can be heard as
a result of the latter.

Such a clear statement of deficient parenting made near the beginning of the
conference establishes an orientation for the rest of the meeting. Lack of parental
control leading to children out of control is the key starting point; it is a point
frequently revisited.

In turn 46, a major contrast is made between the 'caring mother' and 'inadequate
parent', between love and management. Kathy loves her children and they love
her, there is a good relationship and the children are 'attached'. The social worker
draws on psychological notions. Note the use of upgraded formulations ('very
clearly very very attached and very fond of her'). However, the success of Kathy in
establishing this relationship is contrasted with (and it is seen as 'jeopardised' by)
the lack of parental control. Successful parenting appears to require both a
controlling parent and a loving mother, and furthermore the loving/caring aspects
will be undermined by the lack of control and management.

This is an important feature of the depiction of Kathy's moral adequacy. As with
the statements about 'adequate control', it is offered at the beginning of the meeting
as the definitive version of Kathy and the 'inadequate parent/loving mother'

contrast enables any positive version of Kathy's character to be undermined by the negative ones.

As suggested earlier, other contrasts to establish deficient parenting are made without the positive side of the contrast being spelt out. In turns 48 to 51 the concerns about food and diet are outlined by describing the social worker's observations of a poor diet – 'a lot of sweets ehm and other things crisps'. No alternative acceptable diet is described, and listeners are left to complete the contrast. This evaluation is presented as tentative as the social worker sees only some of the children's diet; however synecdoche is a rhetorical device in which a small part is made to stand for the whole (Cockcroft and Cockcroft 1992: 122). It has the same effect as the 'poor parent' formulation and is challenged by Kathy (turn 49). In both formulations, the outcome can be seen in the children's poor behaviour and Ellen's weight gain, however the former is hinted at whilst the latter is established.

Contrasts are a major part of the initial formulation of Kathy as an inadequate parent, as demonstrated in contrasts between her control and adequate parental control, between Kathy as a poor parent and loving mother, between a poor diet and an implicit good diet.

During most of this extract the social worker talks from a personal 'I' perspective. The formulation of Kathy is essentially based on her observations, opinions and evaluations of adequate parenting. There is a widespread use of 'I think', 'I'm concerned', 'my feeling is'. The 'professional vision' (Goodwin 1994) is directly expressed in terms of observations 'I can see' (turn 44) and 'I do observe' (turn 51). However, the 'I' perspective is supported on occasion by linking it to a conversation with Kathy (turn 44) and a view that the social worker observations are only partial on this occasion (turn 51).

We can observe consensual work as other voices are recruited. In turns 47 and 51 there are invitations by the chair and the social worker for other views to be expressed, setting an agenda around which others are encouraged to comment – parenting and diet. There are two recipients for the comment in turn 47: the chair is asking the social worker for a point of view; at the same time, he indicates to the rest of the conference the topics they might consider and how these might be treated. In turn 48, the social worker responds by endorsing the topic widening invitation and rendering the concern with 'food' as a strong collective statement, implying that everyone at the last conference was in agreement about this. In turn 51, as a preface to the social worker's concern about food and diet, there is a specific bid to recruit the views of the home economist, which will support her assessment. Later speakers are being constrained to debate Kathy's parenting in terms of the social worker and chair's formulations.

The speaker who is not recruited however is Kathy. At turn 49 the mother tries to close the debate by saying that the concerns about food raised at the last conference are no longer relevant 'but I've sorted all that out now'. She is quickly rebuffed 'I'll come back to you (.) go on Annie' (turn 50). There are two aspects to this rebuff. It establishes the appropriate occasions on which the client can respond, as well as having the effect of silencing disagreement and thus indicating that legitimate concerns about food remain. This is an example of stage managing:

in the interaction between the chair and the social worker instructions are being tabled to later speakers as to what topics to attend, when to speak, etc. and to emphasise the collectivity of the case conference enterprise.

Being the first major turn, there is emergent cumulative work. As indicated above, the invitation to contribute is in terms of adding to the social worker's observations. Furthermore, the social worker is invited to move from a mere reporting of the decisions and plans at the last meeting to expanding her professional gaze – 'unpack that word parenting'. This move to outline personal observations can be seen as promoting a form of reporting in which layers of opinions and evaluations are built on top of one another, moving from mere facts to deeper insights.

'Not a lack of wanting but a lack of ability'

The social worker is next asked to report on their referral to the Child Guidance team for an assessment of the family. Child Guidance[4] had directed the referral to Norton House, a residential therapeutic unit for families. A family therapist [FT] from Norton House is present. The social worker reads out the reply from Norton House that it is not an appropriate intervention to provide an assessment. Next, the chair invites the family therapist to comment.

Extract 2

62 CH: (to mother) anything else that Annie has said that either you very much agree with or very much disagree with or just comment generally on

63 KM: I I am having problems with their behaviour at the moment

64 CH: so it's the control

65 KM: with Neil more than I am with Ellen (.) Ellen's fine

66 CH: yeah (7)

67 CH: ok thanks – Annie erm made reference to two things one was the letter you've got from Norton House – could we just hear what that says (to FT) and then we'll check with actually

68 SW: right it says *'Harry Shaw'* . well Harry Shaw is from Child Guidance – *'has requested an up-to-date period of residential assessment of the quality of parenting which Ms Malcolm is able to give . her capacity to change and improve the parenting and the relationships within the family . I presented this request to the team who after careful consideration decided that it was not appropriate to offer a further assessment to the family(2) Ms Malcolm and her family were resident at Norton House from 30 April 19__ to 15 June ___ . during her stay Ms Malcolm had an opportunity to work along with the staff to make changes in her parenting skills (.) however Ms Malcolm was unable to generalise the changes or to grasp general concepts of childrearing (.) despite long term outreach work by the child guidance service and family centre . Ms Malcolm failed to meet the children's physical and psychological needs fully . and at present Ms Malcolm's management of her children has deteriorated to the point where the children are now on the child protection register (.) the team has expressed grave concerns about the safety and welfare of the children'* (2) and that was on 24 February

69 CH: ok thanks very much – is there anything you (to FT) want to add to that at all
70 FT: erm just that there were grave concerns expressed about the children but the team as Annie has acknowledged acknowledge the erm close bond between Kathy and the children . Kathy for the children and the children for Kathy . but we are very very concerned about the management of the children
71 CH: erm again I just wonder . the management . is there anything specific that you
72 FT: well just erm I mean when I come to one of these conferences I go back and give a a small report to the team about them . and there's just been continued concerns about what you're saying Kathy . about being unable to manage Neil and erm the children attacking each other and although we (.) I'm very pleased to hear you've been offered a three bedroom house . we did feel that that flat was a contributory factor erm but erm (.) we still feel that there are concerns erm not a lack of wanting to do it but a lack of an ability to do it (.) and so erm that's about as far as we can go
73 CH: (.) ok any comment on that (4) ok thanks …

Before considering professional consensus, it is worth noting the consensual nature of the comment by the mother in an exchange with the chair (turns 63 to 67). Previously, Kathy has strongly defended her attempts to feed and clothe her children adequately. However, in response to the chair's invitation for further comments, she accepts that she has difficulties with controlling the children – 'I I am having problems with their behaviour at the moment' (turn 63). Such a summary statement displays an acceptance of the general drift of the social worker's opening formulation of Kathy's problems in managing the children's behaviour. She highlights Neil's behaviour in particular rather than her own inadequacies, but in turn 65 she does not contradict the chair's comment on 'control'. After a strong bid to challenge the social worker's criticisms about food and clothing, such a comment can be heard as consensual and cumulative, seeking to maintain her position as a cooperative client.

The letter from Child Guidance makes specific assessments of the mother's failure to manage the job of parenting the children and 'her capacity to change and improve the parenting' (turn 68). Examples of her parental failure are outlined – 'unable to generalise the changes', unable to 'grasp general concepts of child rearing', 'failed to meet the children's physical and psychological needs fully'. Again these features are the negative versions of good parenting – change behaviour, understand child rearing, meet physical and psychological needs.

The metaphor of seeing parenting in terms of 'skills' connotes certain methods of behaviour which can be learned and put into practice, and the descriptions of the opportunity to learn from staff and make changes suggests that this was how it was seen. This might be contrasted with 'normal' families who pick up 'parenting skills' from friends or relatives. Although no such direct comparison is made, the general orientation to interventions to teach Kathy imply that she has had deficiencies in her acquisition of such knowledge.

The culmination of the 'deterioration' is proffered as her involvement in the child protection process, although the Child Guidance service is being sought to address this situation – the problem is seen as negating the service. This might be seen as an unusual ending to the refusal of a service – is it being refused because it was offered before and failed or because things are now too serious for child guidance? As will be seen later, this implies an unstated formulation, that the previous intervention did not work and that it is now time to move to a more serious intervention – to remove the children from their mother.

The letter from Child Guidance does not repeat the social worker's contrast between a loving mother and deficit parent, but it is echoed and developed by the family therapist as 'a close bond/concern about management' (turn 70). Note again the use of upgraded terms 'very very concerned' and 'grave concern'.[5] A contrast is also used by the family therapist to illustrate the social and psychological aspects of Kathy's problems. The social surroundings of the flat are seen as 'a contributory factor' but new accommodation will not alter 'the concerns', i.e., the problem remains with Kathy not the flat.

Both the letter and the family therapist make frequent use of 'we' and 'the team' to establish the shared nature of their formulations. In contrast to the social worker, their views are those of a collective. The family therapist portrays the team approach in describing her reporting back, leading to 'continued concerns' from her colleagues (turn 72). The use of an evaluation at the end of the letter is offered as a collective view of the staff at NH. The team had expressed 'grave concern' (turn 70). This echoes the rhetorical device described by Toulmin (1958: 97) as a 'data-warrant-claim'. Here there is ample data about Kathy and a strong warrant, 'grave concern', but no specific claim is made as to what should be done. Listeners are left to recognise the implications.

It has been noted that Kathy accepts the social worker's formulation of deficient parenting to some extent. The family therapist takes the concerns about the children's behaviour further, by upgrading it from Kathy 'unable to manage' to 'the children attacking each other'. She also repeats the social worker's contrast between 'loving mother/inadequate parent' and extends it; the rhetorical is both consensual and cumulative. It is not merely that Kathy is having problems with control, but this is extended to a criticism of Kathy's capabilities, 'not a lack of wanting to do it but a lack of an ability to do it' (turn 72). This is an important addition to the formulation since it is now suggested that the mother is incapable of changing her parenting deficiencies. Norton House has tried and it has not worked, implying any future work is similarly likely to fail. In this way the earlier formulation of the case as one where the mother needs to be helped with her parenting skills is challenged through extending Kathy's deficit character as being beyond help.

In summary, the contributions of the mother, the family therapist and the letter from Child Guidance have revisited and extended the picture of Kathy as a deficient parent. All three contributors have acknowledged the children's behavioural difficulties. The contrasts between normal and Kathy's poor parenting have been extended, the children's behaviour appears more extreme, and most importantly, the mother's deficits are formulated as a result of her inabilities. At the end of this extract, the chair again stresses the consensual nature of the occasion by offering the opportunity for comment.

'Lack of care about her personal self'

The meeting continues with a series of contributions by the teachers, the education welfare officer, health visitor and foster parent, most of which are short, factual, and add little to the mother's character construction. However, one teacher talks at length about Neil's behavioural difficulties at school, which can be heard as further extending the picture of him being 'out of control'. The family centre manager [FCM] is now invited to speak (the centre is located in Goodall):

Extract 3

172 CH: ok Goodall I think are the only people left as major players anything to tell us
173 FCM: it means reiterating . what Sheila's actually keyworking . we actually changed the situation at Christmas with Kathy erm . and we tried to develop a new approach really to see if we could actually erm encourage (.) Katherine to work in a different way erm with Terry and Neil at the centre . so we've given her a different time and different input and a new key worker to see if that would stimulate some change . now I wouldn't question Katherine's love for her children or vice versa . they love mum she loves her children erm . but I would actually pick up on what Norton House was saying . that I don't think it's a case of erm not wanting to to do things for the children . I think it's Katherine's inability to actually see things through erm . we got quite desperate at the centre at Christmas time to actually erm as to what else we could offer erm . having tried a series of different techniques with the children and different approaches . ways of motivating Kathy to get involved and take control . and set limits and boundaries with the children erm (.) I actually would say from what my observations as manager . and I've made sure that I've gone in to see Katherine knowing that Sheila had taken her on as a new key worker . I would say that I have been concerned since Christmas . and this has been shared with Annie and Sheila that I do not see erm her being very motivated as to ehm interacting with Neil and Terry erm (.) and in actual fact I actually question the actual overall feeling of Katherine herself . about how Kathy was feeling and her care for her own her personal self . and that has been talked through with Kathy with Annie and Sheila . so I'd say that I have concerns and I'm really hoping that the house move will actually help . because I feel that we've tried everything that we possibly can within the family centre setting . but Sheila has taken her over in the last twelve weeks

The family centre is described as one of the 'major players' and has offered Kathy both day care and counselling for several years.

As with the family therapist, the family centre manager prefaces her contribution with a 'loving mother/inadequate parent' contrast, similar to the social worker's initial formulation. The social worker in extract 1 had taken three lines of text to describe the positive mother–children relationships with upgraded terms before describing the problems. Similarly, the family therapist in extract 2 presents a positive statement before concerns are expressed. In these formulations the positive version has some credence. The family centre manager, however, begins the formulation in the form of a contrast 'now I wouldn't question Katherine's love for her children or vice versa. they love mum she loves her children erm. but'. The positive statement is cast from the outset in a contrast, with the 'yes/but' format, indicating that it will be downgraded by negative ones.

The family centre manager has repeated and extended the social worker's contrast of good mother/inadequate parent. She now follows this by repeating the same contrast as the family therapist, not 'a case of not wanting' but more Kathy's 'inability to see things through'. The family therapist is explicitly referenced, using similar words. These comments had occurred about 20 minutes earlier in the meeting. The family centre manager then prefaces her own formulation by summarising and appropriating the arguments of other key speakers.

Like the family therapist, the family centre manager begins her contribution by indicating the collective point of view of the team at the family centre. These are in the form of 'we' statements – 'we've given her' and 'we got quite desperate', a spokesperson invested with the authority of the team. However, when the analysis of Kathy's character is made, the personal 'I' is used, drawing on her long association with the family and her 'observation as manager', indicating that she has a special role enabling her to speak with authority. She prefaces her main argument by indicating that her concerns have been shared with the keyworker in the family centre and the social worker.

The family centre manager's formulation extends the character work of the social worker and family therapist and moves it in a different direction. The social worker was juxtaposing the good mother/inadequate parent contrast with the latter aspect in danger of overwhelming the former. The family therapist developed a different contrast of parental failure, not lack of wanting, but her inabilities. The family centre manager moves to question Kathy's personal self-esteem and self-worth. We can see the sequence of this formulation:

> repeat social worker's and family therapist's formulations
>> ⌄ describe new approaches at family centre
>>> ⌄ shared concerns
>>>> ⌄ reached a new, higher level of concern
>>>>> ⌄ Kathy has lost motivation interacting
>>>>>> ⌄ we question Kathy's self-esteem

This formulation makes use of all the character work described so far. The character of Kathy is developed along a set of contrasts, the work is seen as in agreement with other contributors and the final formulation extends the character depiction into more serious areas. The new character assessment is no longer merely an inadequate parent but an inadequate person. The assessment acquires a strong moral overtone.

In summary the family centre manager has repeated, appropriated and extended the increasingly negative character assessment of Kathy. This formulation has built on earlier contributions, made much of the range of interventions and contact with Kathy and her family and produced a strong formulation which points out Kathy's failings in a more pervasive fashion than other contributors. It might be offered as the definitive version of Kathy and has the potential to point towards the need for a new direction in this case, echoing the letter from the child guidance centre that the options for working with this family have become restricted.

Character work as a precursor to decision-making

The case conference has now heard all the evidence and begins the discussion phase. While formally its mandate is to decide whether or not the children should remain on the register (as mentioned earlier), an emerging consensus is that social services should take action to remove the children. Care proceedings are instituted by social services and are therefore technically outside the remit of the case conference. However, the chair cannot ignore such a view altogether, especially as he will seek to maintain consensual decision-making.

It might be assumed at this point that an agreed depiction of Kathy's character has emerged – there is a strong bond between Kathy and her children, she is not managing their care adequately, she has not responded to various interventions, the children's behaviour is getting worse and, as one contributor said, Kathy is 'letting herself go'. The discussion is a long and detailed series of exchanges, but signs of disagreement appear over what should now happen. The chair suggests that further assessment is required but this is challenged by the family therapist. She contends that things just get worse and 'sooner or later we're going to have to make some big decisions', implying that the children may need to be removed.

Extract 4

207 CH: what I would say though is that critically . knowing what happens if big decisions are made . and I guess if if by that's what we are talking about is whether . if Katherine couldn't wasn't seen as able to parent the children adequately would . we'd have to initiate proceedings in the court . for care proceedings . but that's also a huge decision and I guess what we have to live with is that sometimes that does not work happily either . so we need to be very clear I think on the basis of what what we are assessing on at the moment . it doesn't feel to me (.) excuse me . that we've had one concise assessment done which is right up-to-date and could maybe tell us something (.) or indeed that we've actually collected and collated if you see yourselves all as assessing . so so I take your point . I don't think we can just keep rolling either . but it doesn't yet feel that we've got a good basis for that massive decision that maybe we are looking at

208 KM: no matter what I do it seems to be wrong

209 CH: I think it's about trying to turn those things round actually (overlapping)

210 FT: well that's how I feel about it Kathy . you come here to listen to how you haven't done it for every three months . and I find that worrying

211 CH: but I'd I'd turn it around and actually say I've heard lots of things that you clearly have done quite appropriately erm in response to that injury for Terry for

example in . and what I don't hear is that generally erm (.) we are not talking here . I haven't heard about a house which is so erm dirty that that people are saying that those children have to be like out now . or else y'know they're in severe danger of of er their health going down hill and so on and so forth (.) so so I actually think there's lots you are doing to keep it rolling . what I actually think is that network of helping agencies around is struggling to figure out how to to take (the social worker's) views . how to change it for the best as it were once and for all for the future . and that there is a danger that we all begin to run out of energy that that all the systems begin to run out of energy . and that somehow becomes a rationale that something must be done . cos actually I think Katherine's doing an awful lot anyway . and maybe we need to turn it on its head and say what is it more that we can continue to think of to do (.) even though that feels like an uphill struggle . and I certainly think it does for you . I think you've already said (4)

The chair counters the family therapist by acknowledging that Kathy's children might have to be taken into care, however he notes that such action has its own problems: 'sometimes that does not work out happily either' (turn 207). He questions whether there is enough evidence for that 'that massive decision' (turn 207), that is, has a 'last resort situation' been reached, what Emerson (1987: 5) describes as 'the sole course of action remaining'?

A different depiction of Kathy's character is now outlined with a list of positive assessments (turn 211). She responded 'appropriately' for example to Terry's injury. The house isn't 'dirty' and no one is saying that the children should be removed immediately. They are not in imminent 'severe danger' and their 'health (isn't) going down hill'. All these attributes do not suggest the failing parent and person, constructed by earlier speakers. Finally a contrast is made between Kathy's efforts and those of the professionals – Kathy is 'doing lots to keep it rolling' and the 'helping agencies are struggling'.

It is interesting to note the way in which disagreements are managed in a setting in which consensus is expected. The family therapist made a series of extreme case formulations just before this extract – Kathy 'feeling worse and worse and worse' and 'unable to do anything with the children'. Next she suggested that there is 'drift' in decision-making (Rowe and Lambert 1973) with more upgraded devices – 'I don't know many more months', 'sliding on again', 'here we go again'. Whilst this is a strong accusation, it is not aimed at any one professional or agency; nor does it outline a preferred alternative plan.

The chair's formulation similarly draws on consensus whilst disagreeing, and emphasises the need for more assessment. The implication is that there is a difference between an assessment whereby the participants at this conference draw together their opinions and experiences, and 'an Assessment' carried out specifically for the purpose ('one concise assessment done which is right up-to-date' in turn 207).[6] The 'Assessment' is required because of the seriousness of the decision to initiate care proceedings. Whilst the chair also uses the term 'we', on some occasions this refers to the social services department since it is they who will initiate care proceedings and manage the care order (cf. Maitland and Wilson 1987). It is contrasted with 'you' referring to the contribution of other professionals to that assessment, hinting they have a lesser role.

Kathy now realises the critical situation she is in: 'no matter what I do it seems to be wrong' (turn 208) and the family therapist agrees that she is failing (turn 210). The chair reverses the whole direction of the meeting so far by emphasising a number of positive attributes to her care and parenting of the children (turn 211). The alternative depiction undermines the sense of crisis that had been developing, that things are not very serious and perhaps the agencies are overreacting – 'a rationale that something must be done'.

The instruction 'maybe we need to turn it on its head' recommends the professionals to consider the good things rather than concentrate on the negatives, since Kathy is 'doing an awful lot anyway'. Most of this assessment is addressed directly to Kathy with the use of 'you' but aimed at the professionals who are constructed as 'overhearers' (Goffman 1981: 132). In the last statement however, the professionals are being instructed to consider what more they can do. This is a long and complex turn, which appears to 'filibuster' the concerns of the family therapist. A decision has been made and the meeting turns to consider how an assessment might be carried out with no other dissent.

In summary, this extract has shown how the character depiction of Kathy, which has been built through a series of contributions, is re-assessed when the chair senses conflict over decision-making. Positive characteristics of Kathy are highlighted and some blame is directed at the professionals. It is not a complete turnaround in character depiction and interestingly the chair does not return to the 'loving mother' depiction to support his formulation. Rather, the 'other side' of the case is being told, along the lines of 'the glass is half full rather than half empty'. This demonstrates that in order to make decisions, character depiction needs to have some sort of balance with the seriousness of the decision-making. If the established depiction of the failing mother/inadequate person had been accepted by the chair, then the action would have inevitably suggested immediate care proceedings. Nor does the chair say, 'we all agree that the family situation is deteriorating but we'll never get it through the court'. Instead, for the time being, the mother's character is depicted as more complex and not yet irretrievably failing.

Conclusion

This is a long meeting and only certain contributions have been displayed. In particular the mother's contributions have not been examined (Hall and Slembrouck 2001). Our concern has been with the character work done by the professionals and the suggestion that how the mother's character is constructed is central to decision-making in child protection work.

We have seen three processes of character work. First, the character of the mother is established with widespread use of contrasts – good mother/poor parent, not want/not able, cooperative/uncooperative client, adequate/inadequate person, something must be done/doing an awful lot anyway. Second, character assessments are developed consensually, with each professional appearing to agree with the previous one, but then making refinements which hint at slightly different depictions. Third, it is a cumulative process whereby contributors establish their position by building on the assessments of previous speakers. Ultimately, character depictions and evaluations are re-negotiated when decisions are made and courses of action set out. The character assessment informs the decision but it is also informed by it (cf. Garfinkel 1967 on juries' decision-making).

This analysis contributes to two aspects of professional talk and evaluation and suggests that character work is an important mechanism through which these are achieved – categorisation and blame. In the course of the conference, characterisation has been instrumental in shifting the case category from poor parenting to a mother's low self-esteem. The two imply different forms of intervention: for instance, the former would suggest programmes at improving parent skills helping the mother care for her children (in the case analysed here, these have been tried and failed); the latter implies an orientation to a therapeutic programme for the mother and a suggestion that the children may need 'rescuing' (Fox Harding 1997). In terms of the display of accountability, the family problems are located within the mother (not housing, or a child out of control, etc.). She is ultimately held responsible for the problems of the family. Note how in this case there has been little interest in details of the child's injury but considerable concentration on an assessment of the mother's character. At each stage in the three contributions to the case conference which we've analysed, a rather different mother was being talked about: the social worker's version has the mother as loving but lacking in control; for the family therapist she tried to do her best but she was not up to it; the family centre manager sees her as an inadequate person and the chair depicts her as making an effort, despite all the problems. Each characterisation comes with its own specific claim of entitlement to 'ownership of experience and information generally' (Shuman 1993: 136). The social worker claims entitlement by saying 'I've seen'; the family therapist relates to a previous, failed intervention (we've offered this service before and it didn't work) and the family guidance centre manager is referred to by the chair as a 'major player' and invokes 'her observations as manager' suggesting also that she has known the client for a long time. It might have been expected that the entitlement of the family centre manager was stronger. Yet, her point of view does not prevail. This and the different characterisations have not prevented the meeting from appearing to maintain a consensus.

It was noted at the beginning of this chapter that professionals are likely to pay particular attention to their performance in key meetings like child protection conferences. We have seen how speakers appear to agree with one another and to build positions by referring to the formulation of others. It is suggested that professionals could gain from being aware of their own and others contrastive, consensual and cumulative work. Furthermore, key motifs, like 'Kathy loves her children but [. . .]' can help in making a bid for establishing definitive assessments and have a powerful influence on later speakers. In other work, it is noted that formulations or stories which seem to sum up the essence of a character reappear in later documents and contexts (Hall 1997: Chapter 6).

The concern expressed by researchers (Farmer and Owen 1995; Corby *et al.* 1996) that consensus and stage-managing stifle debate in child protection conferences is questioned here. The case conference as an occasion to develop an agreed view is highlighted; however, it does not seem that this could be seen as an example of 'groupthink', where participants aim to establish a version of reality which is a product of the group rather than the individual. Psychologists tend to see such activity as 'sterile' and 'defensive' and the search for unanimity as 'restricting the appraisal of alternative courses of action' (Janis 1982). Here professionals did appear to work within an atmosphere of agreement and consensus, but they can also be seen to fight their corner and promote their professional positions. As suggested above, the versions of the mother formulated by each professional are not necessarily in conflict but have slightly different emphases. Whilst there were few examples of open disagreement, it is also not clear that the participants were necessarily in agreement nor would they leave the meeting with the same view of what happened. To get all professionals together in the same room, does not necessarily lead to joint decision-making and coordinated intervention afterwards. The issue is not necessarily one of a common language. All concerned may have had no problems using common terms like 'grave concern', 'assessments', 'control', etc. The difference can equally reside in the application of the categories and how outcomes of meetings are translated into action scenarios.

5 Negotiating roles in a home visit

Pithouse (1987) has noted 'the invisible nature of social work' as signifying the way in which encounters between professional and client frequently take place away from the public gaze. Unlike the doctor, the teacher, etc., a large amount of the work takes place in the client's home. With home visits, we also move into the least public arenas of social work. The tradition of child welfare social workers visiting the family can be seen along two dimensions: investigative and service-oriented. Part of building a picture of the client is to assess the home environment – how tidy it is, whether there are toys for children, whether it is safe, etc. One of the recommendations of the report of the Climbié Inquiry (Laming 2003: 375) highlights the importance of home visits and the need for them to have a clear purpose:

> **Recommendation 34.** Social workers must not undertake home visits without being clear about the purpose of the visit, the information to be gathered during the course of it, and the steps to be taken if no one is at home. No visits should be undertaken without the social worker concerned checking the information known about the child by other child protection agencies. All visits must be written up on the case file.
>
> (paragraphs 5.108 and 6.606)

In contrast to home visits as a form of inspection, they can also form a service feature of social work, a gesture of outreach towards the client (as in the case studied in this chapter).

A large proportion of the discursive literature on the professions has concentrated on client–professional communication, especially in the medical setting. A review of the literature, particularly concerning social work, has shown that professional–client contact can be considered in terms of several distinctive interactional activities – assessing and diagnosing, assessing eligibility, troubles-telling and advice-giving. Whilst overlapping, these activities highlight different aspects of the professional–client encounter and could be analysed in terms of different frames of reference and activity (see Chapter 2). The first might be seen as the 'diagnostic activity' in which the professional develops and negotiates the client's problem/condition, and it is usually associated with objective/scientific aspects of professional knowledge (e.g. ten Have 1991). The second assesses the client's problems in relation to the service – how does the client qualify for what sort of assistance and support, the 'screening activity' (e.g. Sarangi and Slembrouck 1996 on bureaucratic encounters). The third activity, troubles-telling is particularly associated with the 'counselling activity' of client–professional encounters, in which the clients unburden their problems to the professional (e.g. Jefferson and Lee 1992 on service encounters). The fourth activity, 'advice-giving', is concerned with the professional imparting suggestions for action (e.g. Heritage and Sefi 1992 on health visitors). It is not suggested that these four activities form a neat typology of professional–client encounters but that they suggest rather different orientations to the encounter on the part of the researcher – if they are looked at as troubles-telling, then the diagnostic activity may be underplayed.

From the point of view of this study of child welfare social work in the UK, there is also something missing in this list: the idea of an ongoing helping relationship and, with it, ongoing surveillance. That is, the home visit is often one of an ongoing set of multi-faceted encounters, and it is often surrounded by legislative and bureaucratic considerations. Furthermore, with the promotion of principles like partnership and befriending, the social worker aims (if not necessarily with success) to develop a helping and informal relationship as central to the visit, not merely a polite by-product.

From an interpersonal perspective, the analysis of such encounters requires a sensitivity to unspoken assumptions. That is, we must be aware that it is likely that what is said may be reacted to in terms of what has been said on other occasions and what participants consider is being suggested, if not explicitly stated. For example, in one of the few analyses of social worker–client interviews in the UK, Stenson (1993: 58) argues that an exchange should be considered in terms of 'the unstated but implicit doubt about the client's mothering competence'. That is, what is said is responded to by participants in terms of previous interviews and activities over the children being considered 'at risk'. So that when a mother talks about her worries about her partner's children who are living with his previous partner, the question 'Would you have then [. . .] B hasn't asked you to have them?' is heard as a comment on the problems this would cause her if she was required to take them on. This work will be explored further, but for now we wish to remind the reader of the need for a form of analysis which is both concerned with the nature of the conversational exchanges but also the attribution of contexts (see discussion of frames in Chapter 2).

Another important theme to emerge from the literature is the suggestion that the establishment of categories of clienthood are much less central compared to our discussion of other sites of social work. In the case conference and the policy inter-view chapters, we were particularly concerned with the way in which participants constructed and negotiated categories of clienthood to the extent that 'what type of client is this?' appeared to be the main activity of the encounter. If we can identify and categorise the client then we can make decisions, carry out plans, justify ourselves. In comparison with the work discussed in Chapters 3 and 4 there is much less discussion of categorisation and particularisation. Perhaps in work on assessing eligibility, there is interactional work to enable the participants to attempt to establish the client as a certain sort of person who fits the bureaucratic categories for offering help. For example, Spencer (2001: 162) is interested in the way that clients and social workers negotiate 'biographical particulars of clients' selves for organisational processing'. So, certain kinds of selves are constructed by the clients – 'troubled', 'stranded' and 'trying' – and offered as appropriate for support from the agency. However, the social worker does not necessarily challenge these client self-presentations but instead assesses how far they comply with 'a discourse of rules and resources' of the agency:

> There appears to be a working consensus that obligates social workers to accept the true value of the clients' presented selves, against which a counter-discourse requires counter legitimation.
>
> (Spencer 2001: 171)

In the home visit, the central feature of the interaction may well be to manage the clash of different interactional activities without attempting to construct a definitive, mutually acceptable category. So, while one purpose may well be to make assessments and evaluations of risks to the children in the home for inclusion in later reports, the need to maintain a cooperative and ongoing relationship with the client entails that such an assessment may not be shared with the client in an explicit way.

Similarly, in diagnostic encounters, categories of illness or disability are likely to be raised but the establishment of a shared version of the case is not necessarily the central feature of the interaction. Gill and Maynard (1995: 26) note the way that categories of what sort of developmental disabilities were being suggested by the doctor could be downplayed where parents were thought to be resistant:

> Thus in an environment of uncertainty and possible conflict, clinicians may persuasively portray the appropriate label as one that will solve practical problems, not as one that is necessarily technically correct or that is a pristine, objective reflection of the child's abilities and their diagnostic categories.

As was seen in Chapter 4, in the case conference the client categories were apparently negotiated without any consideration of their implications for ongoing work with the mother. In the analysis that follows then, we will be aware of these two features: that what is said in social work–client home visits is affected by earlier encounters and that categorisation and particularisation are less explicitly the central activity of the encounter.

The lack of direction in the social worker–client interview

It has been noted that there are few discourse studies of social work–client interactions, in particular exploring social work as an ongoing set of encounters concerned with a 'helping relationship'. A key concept that will be used in exploring our data can be attributed to Stenson (1993): indirection. Baldock and

Prior (1981) and Nijnatten *et al.* (2001) also discuss the lack of direction in social worker–client interviews.

Baldock and Prior (1981) compare the nature of social worker-client talk to that of doctor–client talk. They are interested in exploring whether social workers were better at listening and responding to their clients than Byrne and Long found was the case with doctors. They were not disappointed:

> Compared to doctors, even the most unhurried, all the social workers were at all times better listeners, more tolerant of silences and more likely to ask open-ended questions.
>
> (1981: 23)

They also offer an overview of the nature of verbal exchanges in the social work interview. Although not from the discourse analytic perspective, they note the 'conversational' nature of the social work-client interview, particularly compared with the formality of the doctor–patient interaction. The social worker is described as getting the client to talk, playing the role of the listener with the client as storyteller. In one interview the client talks over 80 per cent of the time with most of the social worker's turns consisting of 'yes' and 'um':

> The workers were using the interviews to collect information about the pattern of clients' daily lives and their feelings in order to calculate the danger of their problems getting any worse.
>
> (1981: 30)

However, Baldock and Prior considered that clients were uncertain about the aims of the interview and social workers gave little sense of direction, as evidenced by the difficulty in ending the interview. It was not clear when it was over since the client was not clear about the purpose. The 'non-judgemental stance' also meant that there was a 'purposeful avoidance of disapproval or approval' – there was rarely an expression of surprise:

> The determination not to lecture, admonish or generally 'put down' clients lends the interviews a curiously ramshackle air as the clients ramble on, anything and everything they say being received with the same apparent equanimity.
>
> (1981: 35)

Even so the social workers were considered to have directed the interview and covered the required topics, even if the clients found this difficult to recognise.

The theme of uncertainty and indecision is repeated in two more recent papers on social work–client interviews. First, Stenson (1993) develops the notion of 'indirection' from what Donzelot (1980: 217) calls 'an expert in indecision'. He repeats some of the themes mentioned in Baldock and Prior – the lack of 'social standing and traditional authority', the location of the interview in the home and the promotion of 'friendship models'.

This results in two modes of conversational discourse, by the social worker, what I describe as citizen exchange discourse – talk among *as if* equals – and hierarchical, normalizing discourse. In this discourse the client is incited to adopt the subject position of storyteller.

(1981: 53)

In an analysis of an interview where the social worker and client are discussing the management of debts, apparent differences emerge over some of the client's methods for acquiring money but the social worker declines to openly criticise her:

We can see indirection is a significant feature of the social worker's discourse in this interview. Rejection through withdrawal replaces an open linguistically framed rejection of the client's alternative.

(1981: 65)

The theme of indirection is also reported by van Nijnatten *et al.* (2001) in a study of interviews between parents and family supervisors in The Netherlands. The family supervisor is a social worker who administers a supervision order imposed by the family court where there are child protection concerns, thus a similar designation to the child and family social worker in the UK. Van Nijnatten *et al.* (2001) found that there was 'indirection' in the way that family supervisors were vague about the nature of their legal authority. They used strategies to mask their authority and promoted cooperation with the parents to protect the child. For example, when outlining her role to parents:

The family supervisor formulates her authority as 'something might be said' and 'it could perhaps happen quite once in a while'. The use of interjections like 'might', 'would' and 'could perhaps' makes her utterances indirect.

(2001: 712)

In another case, the option of placement in care is presented so indirectly that it seems to be a highly unlikely intervention. Van Nijnatten *et al.* (2001: 717) are critical of such practices, seeing these as a lack of skill in confronting clients and overemphasising cooperation.

These studies all report 'indirection' and lack of clarity in social work–client interviews but look to wider explanations – e.g. poor practice, lack of skill, the disguised nature of disciplinary power. It assumes that there is a more 'direct' form of social worker–client interaction which is (more or less) easily distinguished but is being avoided. Social workers, compared to, say, doctors, do not have clearly defined roles and expectations which the clients recognise and they do little in their communication to clarify roles and expectations . For Stenson (1993) the lack of clarity is evident in the way in which the social worker's views of the client's deficiencies and behaviour are not made explicit. Instead disapproval is hinted at – 'you aren't taking on more children, given your present coping problems' – or actions are not supported. For van Nijnatten *et al.* (2001) the indirection is apparent in the lack of a clear explanation of the social worker's role and authority. Both client identities and social worker identities are vague, it is not clear how the client is being constructed, what is expected of them and how authorities might act to control their deficiencies.

Using a discourse analytic approach we have the opportunity to move in the opposite direction, to look to a more detailed examination of how 'indirection' is constructed and managed. That is, to look at its dynamics rather than its origins. Furthermore, this notion of 'indirection' provides us with an arena to explore whether or not this constitutes an apparent lack of categorisation behaviour mentioned above, in contrast to other sites of social work. Are the social workers and clients avoiding the clarification of categories of clienthood and professional identity? An alternative approach is to explore how this 'indirection' might better be seen as the extension of the negotiation and particularisation of identity categories. In Chapter 3, we have discussed the way in which categorisation works to both identify what sort of person or problem this is: it is a case of a child sex abuser. We have also noted that such work may also involve particularising the category (Billig 1985): this is a child abuser who supports his family. Thus it is suggested that 'indirection' might be seen as an extension of particularisation. That is, rather than approach such interactional work as a failure to establish categories, we might see 'indirection' as the negotiation of the particulars around the category, without making the category the focus of the interaction.

Stenson's work points in this direction through his discussion of the case of the hostile client (1993: 57–67). He introduces the case through a categorisation, 'a mother whose children are on the 'at risk' register and who have chronic debts', and suggests that the interview takes place, with this category not made explicit but hinted at. The question by the social worker, 'Would you have them? (1.0) B, hasn't asked you to have them?', re-constructs and negotiates the category of mother:

> Now, within this particular setting, this question cannot be innocent, given that both parties know that the client's mothering competence with her own, let alone anyone else's children, is the subject of scrutiny. Yet, significantly, at the point the client does not make explicit reference to the topic of this scrutiny, which is implied in the social worker's turn.
>
> (1993: 59)

He is suggesting that both parties are aware of the work that this question is doing, given the 'microculture' which has been built up over time between the client and social workers. Both know that the context of the interview is the mother's competence and, although this question is 'ambiguous', it contributes to both the status of her clienthood and its consequences. Such vagueness, we suggest, is categorisation at work. Rather than the main activity of the encounter being the establishment of the category, mothering competence, the social worker and client debate the particulars and the properties of the category, e.g. taking on other children. How far the negotiation of particulars establishes or relativises the overall category is of course a matter for detailed analysis.

Analysing a home visit

Our analysis is based on a brief interview between a social worker and a mother (Danielle Moynahan) of three children (1 girl, Chrissie, and 2 boys, Nathan and Gerry). Danielle, who lives in a London borough, has been divorced from the father of these children and it came to light subsequently that the father had been sexually abusing the daughter. Court orders have been made concerning the mother's custody of the children and the father's contact with them, which has changed since the discovery of the abuse. There is however concern about how the family are now coping and an order has been made by the court to ensure that the family are supported and the contact arrangements monitored. This social worker is fairly new to the case and there have been several professionals previously involved in the high profile events of the court case and custody/contact proceedings. This particular visit centres around the father's contact visits with the boys.

Our analysis will focus on how the client and social worker negotiate statuses of the clienthood and social work: what sort of client is Danielle and what constitutes social work support in relation to her client status? In line with the literature, which notes that notions of client and social worker are vague (in comparison with doctor–patient or teacher–student), we will explore how such statuses are negotiated during the interview through legitimation and alignment: (1) how does the client construct herself and the other members of the family as particular client types, (2) how does she construct social work as a profession both in contrast to other social workers and in response to her problem and, (3) how does the social worker respond to the formulation of the father as a problem and (4) how does the social worker handle what appears to be a challenge to the legitimacy of her professional role.

Delineating the family

Our data begin with the opening of the exchanges of the home visit. The social worker invites an update.

Extract 1

01 SW: how how're the boys Danielle just

02 DM: erm

03 SW: just give me an update (indistinct, speech tails off)

04 DM: (.) Nathan was a bit upset when he came back the other day erm

05 SW: from contact (.) is that with (father)

06 DM: erm yeah he said erm that he was upset because his dad wouldn't listen to him
. he's told him that he'd buy him a complete school uniform

07 SW: hmm

08 DM: and he got upset because he insisted on buying him a (laugh) pair of school
trousers and Nathan didn't want these particular school trousers

09 SW: hmm

10 DM: and he must've carried on saying that he didn't want it and he got upset because his dad wouldn't listen to him and he said you've got to have proper school trousers erm (.) and the other

11 SW: was that on Saturday Danielle

12 DM: yeah that was on the Saturday

13 SW: right

14 DM: and the other little thing was when he cooked him a dinner he said that he wanted (laugh) mushrooms and his dad said you don't like mushrooms and Nathan said yes I do so but apart from that he was ok

The social worker's opening question, which is part of the procedural routine of inviting the client to tell her story (Baldock and Prior 1981), asks the mother to assess the children's well-being. Whilst such a question is an invitation to tell a story, it also puts Danielle in the position of being able to speak about her children. The mother accepts such a role, even before the social worker has finished speaking. At turn 02 she interrupts the social worker, resulting in the social worker's speech tailing off in turn 03. There is a short pause before Danielle starts at turn 04 further establishing her right to speak on this topic.

The social worker takes the pause at the end of turn 04 to locate and perhaps facilitate the storytelling. This is done co-constructively as Danielle raises the problem 'Nathan was a bit upset' and the social worker locates the source of the problem 'from contact . . . with father'. Although Danielle begins by talking about Nathan's state of mind (implying a cause of distress), it is the social worker who locates the source of his distress in the institutionalised category of 'contact'. Given that the social worker correctly interprets 'he came back' as meaning 'from contact . . . with father', it can be anticipated that this shared construction of the source of trouble was established before this interview.

In turns 06 to 10 Danielle tells a story of how Nathan got upset. It is a complete story (Labov and Waletzky 1967) with an abstract (he was upset because his father wouldn't listen to him), orientation (dad promised a school uniform), complication (only bought him trousers and Nathan didn't want these trousers), resolution (father insisted on these trousers), and evaluation (father wouldn't listen to him). Note how the story is prefaced and concluded by Nathan saying that his father was not listening to him, using the child's reported speech to condemn the father. In this way, the criticism is coming from the child not Danielle herself, giving it evidential status (Smith 1993). There is laughter at one point as if to show the pettiness of the situation. A similar story follows at turn 14 about the father insisting that Nathan did not eat mushrooms, also with a laugh to signify Danielle's disapproval of her husband's behaviour. Danielle's storytelling is completed with a coda ending at line 14, 'apart from that he was ok'. The social worker encourages the storytelling with appropriate backchannel 'hmm' and questions which display her knowledge of contact arrangements – 'was that on Saturday'.

Already in this opening sequence, we see a differentiation between the children and the father as elements of the family, the first sensitive and dependent and the second insensitive and excluded. Notice that Danielle's concern here is with a deficient father (as opposed to, say, an inconsiderate husband). In as much as the father is portrayed as not listening to his son, the mother presents herself as sensitive to the child's point of view. We can observe that both the mother and the social worker are constructing Danielle as a competent parent. First, she is given and accepts the task of assessing the boys' well-being. Second, she depicts herself in contrast to the insensitive father. In doing so a preferred family set-up is (re)established – the mother and her children with the insensitive father excluded. There is alignment between the mother and the social worker: the mother is established as the legitimate spokesperson for the family and a preferred family set-up is being jointly re-visited.

Outside help

In the next set of exchanges the problem is redefined, once again by Danielle:

Extract 2

15 SW: right and did he keep his distance when he dropped the boys off
16 DM: yeah
17 SW: or so he didn't come in
18 DM: no
19 SW: and try and talk to you
20 DM: no
21 SW: and threaten you so that's stopped a bit since before Christmas
22 DM: erm no monday last monday he brought the boys back and Gerry had lost his front door key and I went to the door to open it and he shouted out I love you (.)
23 SW: to you not to (overlapping)
24 DM: yeah to me and then the boys came in and Nathan said dad said that you'll want us (.) that you would like to come swimming with us and I said you know that I'm not going out with you and daddy and they both got upset (-)
25 SW: hmm
26 DM Gerry said dad's only trying to be friendly
27 SW: hmm
28 DM: so I've got to get some (.) outside help with this I think erm
29 SW: what what sort of outside help Danielle is that
30 DM: (.) just advice how I can explain to them because they don't
31 SW: yeah
32 DM: seem to understand

In Extract 2 the social worker attempts to explore if there is still a problem of a threat to Danielle herself. Again presumably alluding to previous interviews, the social worker asks about another set of concerns – did the father keep his distance (turn 15), come in and talk (turn 17–19) and threaten her (turn 21). Note the form of the list with the last three negative items as an escalating three-part list

(Jefferson 1990). Such a set of possible concerns is offered in the form of a contrast device (Smith 1993) – the insensitivity towards the boys as opposed to the threat to the mother, with a suggestion that whilst one set of problems remains the same, perhaps another set has become less of a concern.

The mother initially concurs with this contrast, perhaps because it would mean providing evidence to overturn each of the negatives. However she challenges the summary statement that it is better than before Christmas (turn 21). From turn 22 to 28 Danielle tells another story of continuing concerns about the father. First, in terms of the threat to Danielle, the father comes to the door and shouts 'I love you'. The social worker checks that this remark is aimed at the mother, again using the negative 'not to . . .' This statement of apparent endearment is interpreted by both parties as a threat to Danielle, displaying the shared understanding of Danielle and the social worker. Note how a pause at the end of turn 24 is used to recruit alignment from the social worker. Second, Danielle extends the threat by relating how the boys have started to take on the father's bid for an alternative family set-up. They concur with the suggestion to go swimming, a family outing depicting a version of the family as the children and both parents. Note how the father is now depicted as sly, since he tells the boys that the swimming invitation is the mother's suggestion. This is set up as a major source of trouble to Danielle, with the boys' getting 'upset' and Gerry offering a strong alternative formulation of family relations, again using reported speech (turn 26).

Whilst the social worker provides support in the form of backchannelling, there is no direct alignment with this new set of concerns, (for example, 'this must be hard to handle'). Without such a summary statement Danielle moves to reconfigure the problem as serious enough to require 'outside help' (turn 28) which will enable her to communicate the complexity of the situation to the boys (turn 30). In other words, she needs to have access to a professional discourse – a mode of talk, which will enable her to clear up any misunderstanding and help her undermine the alternative family set-up which the boys have taken on from the father. Again note the pause before she uses the term 'outside help' giving it greater credence. Here we see a client constructing herself as wanting to take initiative. Such a controlling mode is possible only if the mother is able to establish herself as able to assess her children's needs and define the preferred family set-up and as someone who can identify the appropriate support. She is thereby making a bid for professional expertise.

The social worker does not concur with this formulation and the question at turn 29, 'what sort of outside help Danielle, is that' can be heard as a challenge. This can be observed in the way that the phrase 'outside help' is repeated, appearing to problematise the notion, or at least querying it. Furthermore, on previous occasions where the social worker asked a question, it was to elicit more information to amplify an emerging story. Here, however, Danielle has reached the end of her formulation with a summary statement at turn 28. The social worker provides no support for this conclusion and the implication of the question is that the conclusion does not follow from the formulation. Also that the social worker's emphatic repetition of her name, Danielle, appears to reaffirm her client status.

In this exchange, then, Danielle has sought further legitimation for her qualifications to locate the needs of her family, to identify threats and to establish the preferred family set-up. She is making a bid to not only make specific the concerns but to locate the appropriate response. In terms of gaining the alignment of the social worker, she has been able to resist any notion that the threats from the father have changed. Furthermore, she has established that these threats have led to 'upsets' in the family that challenge the preferred family set-up. However, she has not been able to recruit the social worker's support for the preferred remedy.

Appropriate help

With the mother having finished her formulation, the social worker now assumes the position of main speaker. She takes Danielle's assessment of the problem and preferred solution and appropriates it to re-establish her social work role in this case. As far as the social worker is concerned, she is there to give the sort of advice which the mother wants and seeks to establish that she is that 'outside help'. However, in doing so, she undermines Danielle's bid for access to a professional mode of talk.

Extract 3

33 SW: yeah I guess I mean that's one of the things that I I see the boys once a fortnight I should be trying to help them with finding out what they find difficult

34 DM: yeah

35 SW: about coming back and going to dad's cos

36 DM: yeah

37 SW: all children find that very difficult erm particularly when they

38 DM: and really (overlapping)

39 SW: live with one parent and see another

40 DM: how best I can cope with it so I don't say the wrong things that's what I'm

41 SW: yeah

42 DM: worried about erm

43 SW: cos Nathan seems to be the one that is struggling a bit with it isn't he

44 DM: yes

45 SW: yeah he's cos he's younger than Gerry and I think he's the one that really wanted contact wasn't he

46 DM: yes he keeps asking me well he keeps saying that he doesn't like social workers he doesn't like me (.) for the reason that I'm stopping him from going to sleep over his dad's flat though he's never said anything like this before so whether anything's been sort of

47 SW: (overlapping) ok so perhaps that's what I'll do with them next week when I come to see them I'll have a long talk with both of them about what they understand by what the court ordered and what (court social worker) had spent a lot of time talking to them about cos I've only really seen them on two occasions cos I'm quite new to the case

Turn 33 marks an important shift. The social worker begins with apparent agreement ('yeah') followed by a triple hedge ('I guess I mean that's one of the things') before alluding to the two-weekly meetings as the occasion which indicates that it is part of her brief to counsel the boys on these matters. Note in particular the use of 'should' in turn 33 to denote that it is incumbent on the social worker to help the boys in this way. The social worker seeks legitimation by displaying both her familiarity with this type of situation (turn 37) and her knowledge of the particular needs of the boys (turn 43). Despite initially agreeing with the social worker (turns 34 and 36), the mother begins to talk across the social worker, re-stating her earlier formulation. It is Danielle herself who needs help to both manage the whole situation ('how best I can cope with it') and to be equipped with an appropriate language ('so I don't say the wrong things' turn 40). This draws on notions of self-help and empowerment, in contrast to the social worker's direct approach, which invokes expert systems.

Again the social worker expresses apparent agreement with Danielle, but does not specifically support the formulation of self-help. Instead the social worker moves to another topic of the boys' particular needs and in showing her knowledge of Nathan's needs, asks for alignment ('isn't he' (turn 43) and 'wasn't he' (turn 45)). In turn 46, Danielle provides extra information which supports the social worker's concerns about Nathan, but uses the formulation to hint at problems associated with social work intervention, 'he keeps saying that he doesn't like social workers'. This challenge is then softened to depict a more general complaint 'he doesn't like me', since both are stopping him from sleeping at his father's flat and this is a recent occurrence.

In turn 47 the social worker interrupts Danielle's turn to provide a definite statement of what should now happen and in doing so, she firmly establishes herself as the appropriate help for the boys. She provides a detailed description of her intentions – have a long talk, examine what they understand about the court order, take on the role of the previous social worker.

Expressions such as 'I should be trying to help', 'that's what I'll do', 'I'll have a long talk', appear to be deterministic, in the form of an instruction, rather than voluntaristic, seeking an invitation (e.g., 'If you like I could talk to the boys'). The assumption here is that the social worker is better equipped than the mother to explain things to the children. The social worker sees her role as both supporting Danielle and talking to the children – rather than allowing Danielle to manage the children on her own. This, of course, is a very powerful appeal to a model of intervention in which the 'professional knows best'. In this case, the mother's right to produce a formulation of the circumstances is reduced to stating the problem but not directing the solution.

In summary, legitimacy has shifted from the mother depicting herself as assessing family needs and the preferred family set-up to the social worker establishing her role as the appropriate help in this case and outlining the future course of that help. Whilst there has been alignment in terms of the nature of the problem, potential disagreement about the appropriate help has been sidestepped by talking across one another. In terms of 'indirection' we have seen the social worker as very active, in both exploring the mother's stories and formulations and imposing her own formulations on the situation, which is achieved by undermining the mother's bid for control. Furthermore, client categories and social work roles have been negotiated and (re)established. The mother is both a competent parent in terms of understanding her children's needs and defining the preferred family set-up. The father is deficient and dangerous: insensitive to the children, threatening towards Danielle and attempting to undermine the preferred family set-up. The boys are not coping well, they challenge present arrangements and need help. The social worker has imposed herself as the appropriate help in terms of counselling the boys. This has been accomplished without any arguments, although subtle and unexplored disagreements have been sidestepped.

'It's still not running smoothly is it?'

In the next exchanges, we see the mother and the social worker reach an explicit alignment over the state of affairs.

Extract 4

48 DM: (overlapping) yeah Gerry said don't blame me mum but dad's coming to collect us on your birthday which is on a Sunday night the day which he shouldn't see them ehm they've got grading at their karate club and Gerry said don't blame me mum but dad's going to bring you a birthday present I don't know why he said but ehm

49 SW: hmm

50 DM: I sense trouble on that particular night

51 SW: (overlapping) has he kept to the times because I know you had some difficulty about him coming back with some mates and I know he has mucked you around with days saying he will take them out when it is not his day to do that

52 DM: ehm no he has kept to the Friday night that he said

53 SW: right and the Saturday

54 DM: and this Sunday coming up

55 SW: right

56 DM: because of the gradings at the karate club

57 SW: so he sees them on Tuesday and Saturday

58 DM: on Monday and Saturday

59 SW: Monday evening but he has changed that a bit in the last two weeks

60 DM: yeah

61 SW: yeah

62 DM: (cough)

63 SW: So it's it's still not running very smoothly is it

64 DM: No

65 SW: No

66 DM: Not really

In this series of exchanges we can see the social worker and Danielle moving to a marked explicit alignment. At the end of the previous extract, the social worker has taken a strong position to assert her role and sense of direction in the case – she will talk to the boys and establish herself as the site of counselling and 'outside help'. This formulation is not acknowledged by Danielle (for example, 'oh that would be helpful'). Instead she talks over the social worker's turn and begins a new story about Gerry, the older boy (turn 48). That it is about the older boy can be heard to extend the nature of the concerns since in the previous extract only Nathan was identified as a concern. The way in which Gerry's words are presented further intensify the sense of threat. The use of reported speech again takes the listener directly into the encounter. Gerry is heard to highlight the unease 'don't blame me mum', which prefaces the revelation about the father's visit: he senses why this is a worry. The father is coming on a Sunday night when he should not. After the explanation of karate grading, Gerry's words are repeated with the added threat of a birthday present. Gerry is heard as identifying a potential threat in similar terms to the sources of worry already identified by Danielle.

The mother appears to downplay Gerry's intentions ('I don't know why he said that'), making it clear that she cannot be heard to be encouraging such a formulation. His story appears to come from nowhere nor does she explain how she responded to it: it is enough that it is left to hang in the air. She now quickly moves to use the story to make clear its significance ('I sense trouble on that particular night' turn 50). Such a strong statement of impending threat intensifies the nature of the threat to the family and resists the social worker's earlier attempt to downplay its extent at turn 21. However, this strong statement is not acknowledged by the social worker and, like Danielle at turn 48, the social worker talks over Danielle's alarm.

Another aspect of contact arrangements is introduced by the social worker: whether the father is sticking to the agreed contact arrangements. Whilst this is an opportunity to further condemn the father, Danielle downplays this problem. He is generally sticking to the correct days. The social worker appears a little confused by which days these are (turns 52–59). However, the mother notes that it has changed for particular events (turn 54), although she does not appear to see this in itself as a problem. After a cough by the mother that functions as a pause, the social worker provides an overall assessment of the current state of affairs: 'it's still not running very smoothly is it' (turn 63). This is acknowledged by both speakers (turns 64–66).

This series of exchanges at the beginning of a social work interview has essentially been concerned with negotiating what is the current state of affairs or what sort of case is this? The final alignment that 'it's not going smoothly' can be seen as the culmination of a series of negotiations over social work roles, the right to assess the boys' well-being, contact arrangements, threats to the family and that intra-familial communication is under strain. However, each of these topics has been raised but not necessarily resulted in a specific acknowledgement of agreement and hence alignment. The boys' distress has been raised but there has been disagreement as to how it should be handled. The contact arrangements are working well but in some respects they are not. The threats to Danielle have been maintained but in other ways the situation has improved. The effects on the intra-family communication are acknowledged but there is no agreement about how it should be handled. The social work role is being negotiated but not necessarily accepted. The mother has a right of talk about her family but not to decide on the appropriate service.

At the same time, this series of exchanges at the beginning of a home visit displays negotiation over the character of the father. Both speakers have indicated that he is a source of threat to the family and negotiated the particulars. Neither party refers to the father's status as a child sex offender, but there are allusions to the court restrictions (turns 15–19 in Extract 2). Apart from that, it is his current behaviour and the consequences of the contact arrangements that are under consideration. The question is what degree of disruption does he cause to the family? In extract 1 the mother depicts him as insensitive to the boys, but this episode is finished with a low level threat, 'apart from that he was ok'. The second extract is concerned with how far he is a threat to Danielle herself which is acknowledged and then transfers to the way he is disrupting the intra-family relations. In the third extract, the effects on Nathan are discussed and in extract four the threat is seen from Gerry's point of view. At each point the level of threat is negotiated and slightly increased. So that in the final extract, Danielle can 'sense trouble' (turn 50) and the social worker sums up that 'things are not running smoothly' (turn 63).

'Both of them said they didn't want it did they'

In the last extract, it appears that agreement has been reached about the nature of the family's problems. Some minutes later the means of tackling these problems still remains at issue.

Extract 5

101 DM: what's bothering is the fact that Nathan keeps saying when can I go and see their daddy's flat

102 SW: hmm yeah and I think you've got

103 DM: because I don't know whether that's been whether it's been put into his mind or whether he's naturally wanting to go and stay at his flat I know he doesn't want to come back and he keeps saying that he'd like to go and live with his dad later

104 SW: I guess it's quite difficult for him to understand why why he can't go if he's had that before and he's been overnight when y'know living here or being with somebody for seven days a week and then suddenly to be told well no you can't stay overnight and Nathan was from reading about the notes I mean Nathan didn't really have any idea about some of of the allegations made by the girls

105 DM: no if I say anything if he says well why don't you love daddy anymore and I try to explain he's then saying I know daddy touched Chrissie in that place but I still love him and why don't you take him back so he just can't put the two together and understand so

106 SW: ok well I see then next I'll have a good talk with them about what they understand about and what they can

107 DM: which is why I was wondered whether counselling would benefit them

108	SW:	but they didn't want it did they they you all went along to family therapy didn't you and both of them said they
109	DM:	hmm
110	SW:	didn't want to continue that I mean it could be that they'll
111	DM:	yeah
112	SW:	come back to that a later point and say yes erm to it if it's offered again but I mean Gerry fairly adamant about that isn't he
113	DM:	he is yeah
114	SW:	erm and said on one occasion when I spoke to him that he'd rather just talk to somebody in an informal way rather than go off to family therapy

The mother continues to highlight the difficulty that the boys have in understanding the current family arrangements. To the extent that Nathan wants to go and live with his father later and makes a real bid towards re-establishing the original family. In turn 104, the social worker continues to empathise with the mother's formulation. In her next turn (turn 106), she takes the problem off the mother by offering 'I'll have a good talk with them about what they understand about and what they can'. This turn is responded to by Danielle continuing her unfinished previous turn 'which is why I wondered whether counselling would benefit them'. This revisits the earlier problem of negotiating the appropriate roles of client and social worker. In extract 2, the mother was seeking a professional voice and inviting 'external help' to deal with the problem. Here she is requesting counselling for the boys, a different form of outside help. Similarly, in extract 2, the social worker reformulated the mother's request as help she could offer. Here (turn 108 and 110) she appropriates the request for counselling so as to undermine it by casting it not only in terms of an earlier failed intervention of family therapy but also through the point of view of the children's whose speech is being reported in support of her claim: 'both of them said they didn't want it did they'. Finally, the social worker, in turn 114, uses private knowledge of her meetings with Gerry to establish that her support fits the bill: 'he'd rather just talk to somebody in an informal way rather than go off to family therapy'. Note how family therapy is constructed in a distant way 'go off to' whereas her contact with Gerry is 'informal talk'.

'So really I'd have to go to you to ask'

Toward the end of the interview, Danielle expresses concern about the father's continuing threats and where she might turn for support. If the father continues to cause problems how can she get help to try to control him? The social worker says that if he 'blatantly breaks the contact arrangements' she must go back to court. She then points out that the route to court is via herself since there is a court order in operation. However, this information is provided in an indirect way:

Extract 6

211	SW:	(previous social worker from the court) will be at the conference hopefully she'll get an invitation but what she did just before Christmas was to actually

say that she wouldn't be working on the case anymore because the Family
Assistance Order had been granted in our name the local authority's
212 DM: oh its has I didn't know
213 SW: so that it had to be monitored by a social worker from from our office erm
and (previous social worker) did all the submitting of the reports to to get the
contact arrangements in the first place
214 DM: so really I'd have to go to you to ask
215 SW: well you'll have to first of all

This is the only time the order has been mentioned in the interview. Rather like
the supervision order discussed by van Nijnatten *et al.* (2001), its details are not
made explicit. Instead, it is used by the social worker at this stage to further establish
her role. Note the indirect way in which the authority vested in the order is
portrayed. The order is granted 'in our name, the local authority' and it is monitored
by a 'social worker from our office'. It is Danielle who infers the implications: 'so
really I'd have to go to you to ask'. The social worker seems most reluctant to be
explicit about how the court order prescribes her role.

Conclusion

In summary, it was suggested at the beginning of this analysis that the 'indirection'
or vagueness observed in social worker–client communication was not necessarily
the result of a lack of control over the interaction but has more to do with the
negotiation of particulars around the case category. Without specifying the precise
nature of the client status or social work role, the social worker and the client were
centrally concerned with negotiating the nature of the social work but this
negotiation takes place in terms of a concern for the particulars of the case. The
particulars centred on the threats which the father poses, the management of the
contact, the effects on the boys and the instability this created for the mother.
Whilst there was no direct debate of the mother's capacities it was clear that
she was treated as a competent mother who can assess the children's needs and
articulates a need to manage the threats to the family. Her competence as a mother
is never questioned and she is treated as a 'spokesperson' for the family. However,
she is not allowed to become the 'author' of the intervention needed to meet these
problems. Similarly, whilst the social worker's specific role and tasks were not
explicitly debated, there are instances in the interaction where implicit disagreement over her role takes centre stage. The mother appears reluctant to rely on the
social worker as the primary provider of helping services to the family. The social
worker redirects the mother's voiced needs in terms of her services to the boys: the
message is that she is here for the children.

Especially in areas of social work where there is uncertainty about the various
obligations and responsibilities on each side, the mandate which the social workers
brings to a home situation needs to be enacted and negotiated. As we have
seen, positions are put forward, rebuffed, imposed, and a measure of alignment is
established. In this, tension is not necessarily resolved, but a working agreement

is established for the time being, one which is always potentially open to revision, change, etc. Aronsson (1998) uses the metaphor of 'social choreography' for this: such behaviour can be seen in terms of negotiation over role identities (Widdicombe and Wooffit 1995). While an uneasy alignment might be achieved through interaction, at key points the social worker imposes her authority (e.g., denies a particular service, and, in doing so, establishes limitations on the role of the mother by specifying her own intervention, or, further on in the interview, establishes herself as the obligatory channel to continue to manage the father, if necessary, through the court, etc.).

In Chapter 3, we have noted the importance of narrative as a feature of accounting. Here, short narratives are evident as illustrative of positions or formulations, for instance, the mother's description of the contact visit. Narrative, however, is not an overall organising feature of the encounter. Similarly, categorisation, which was the mainstay of Chapter 4, is here backgrounded and remains unresolved. Accountability, however, has been recognisable in the establishment of roles and responsibilities. The social worker is establishing a helping relationship while controlling access to services. The client is concerned to display an identity of a competent parent but equally wanting access to services. Both are attempting to construct defensible and workable role identities. To this extent, it might be expected that social worker and client avoid explicit argumentation over role definitions and instead choose to hint at appropriate expectations for mother and social worker. In contrast to Laming's (2003) concern that social workers' home visits in child protection cases must be more purposeful, we have seen how in more service-oriented visits there is a greater range of activities at work. Any expectations that home visits must have a clear purpose are bound to be limited in scope when set in the context of the careful negotiation involved in the development of a helping relationship between social worker and client.

6   Reporting events in case notes

13–09

(Area manager) phoned (unit manager) at (children's home). Had received a letter from (hospital) describing interview with (mother) the previous Sunday and examination of (child's) broken nose. He was v concerned about (father) being at the home and the injury to (child). I phoned (social worker manager) at hospital + asked him to get information for me as hosp had still not properly informed us of the incident. (Doctor) phoned me she repeated the information given in her letter to (unit manager). There could be no doubt that (mother) had described the incident as accidental caused by her husband. I asked whether the injury was consistent with the explanation especially being caused by a fall downstairs. She said the break could only be caused by excessive force and of severe blow. I said I would be informing the police as I said I thought it should be investigated and she agreed. Phone call from team leader at hospital. His (unclear) of the emergency was not the same as (Doctor) had said to be and did not even mention the broken nose. He agreed to ask police to investigate.

This is a typical entry taken from a social work case record concerning a young mother, Janice Wilkinson, with four children, who has been living together with the father of the children for about eight years. In a nutshell, the eldest child is already in care and was visiting the family in the weekend when the alleged 'broken nose' incident happened. The father is the suspect: he is considered violent and a potential threat to the other three children. He has been ordered by the court to stay away from the family, but the mother disregards this injunction and allows him to see the children on a regular basis. This results in a decision by the social services to remove the other three children with the help of police. The mother contests this decision and the case comes to court. The entries in the case record we focus on in this chapter span over a period of two weeks, leading to the court decision that the children should return home.[1]

There are several features in the recorded entry which attract our attention. A series of past actions are reported (Area manager phoned, I asked, he agreed, etc,); some events are highlighted for further clarification in the near future (e.g., to get information from hospital, to confirm if the incident is accidental or caused by 'excessive force and of severe blow'); and some tentative assessments are hinted ('the break could only be caused by excessive force'). Reference is made to the need for objective evaluation – whether the injury was caused by a fall as opposed to the injury being caused by excessive force, the latter implying possible identification of the perpetrator. The focus of attention is the child's broken nose, although the team leader at the hospital did not even mention the incident. The spotlight falls on the father of the children as the potential perpetrator. But while the identity of the perpetrator is being established through proper investigation, swift action is needed as there is concern about the safety of the other children. This prompts the social worker to contact the police – and through this to keep away from any future blaming for lapses. We get a sense that it is not just an exercise in reporting actions and events, but how an action or event becomes the basis for further investigation. The plot as it unfolds appears complex, full of voices, events and actions. A network of professionals is involved in putting the puzzle pieces together. There are different colleagues from within the social work department, the social worker from the hospital, the doctor, police.

In terms of linguistic features, we notice that the entry is based on both prior talk (telephone conversations) and text (a letter). The origin of most entries in case records lies in spoken interaction. These mainly happen to be phone calls and various face-to-face encounters, as we can see above. The gist of a phone call is entered as 'I phoned . . .', 'I informed . . .'. At times, parts of the case record come across as reconstructed dialogues to give the accounts an authentic and evidential status. It also suggests that a particular perspective – and hence a particular form of accountability – is being established. Elsewhere (Hall *et al.* 1997b) we have analysed in detail an interview with the social worker involved in this case, with a particular focus on which voices become silenced and how the social worker attempts to bring about a preferred state of affairs by keeping the father away from the scene. Such an attempt is routinely foiled by the mother as and when she allows the father access to the children. As we will see, the social work perspective enshrined in the case record will later be challenged by the mother's story.

In this chapter we shall examine closely case records as a crucial site of social work along the general themes of categorisation and accounting practices, i.e., the nature and function of social work files and the overarching circumstances that surround the activity of record keeping. To what extent are case records the professional/institutional equivalent of personal diaries, consisting of self-reports and to what extent are they accountable reports of justifiable professional action which may be presented in court or other evaluative arenas, even in public inquiries? While case notes do provide a documentation of multi-agency networks and displays of a division of labour between professionals, the recent trend towards documentary practices being made electronically available to other agencies raises issues of translation, completeness and anticipated readerships.

Keeping records about clients is a routine professional activity in many institutional sites (Wheeler 1969; Weed 1971; Raffel 1979): education, health, police, etc. They are institutional requirements and are a professional resource. It is through such record-keeping that professionals across institutions build and manage cases of intervention. However, what goes into case records and what is left out is based on professional judgement, although increasingly checklists, procedures and guidelines are directing the nature of recording. Each profession develops its own way of constructing and using case records. Social work records are inevitably different from medical or police case records.

Coherence in a case record is not given but arrived at through specific inferencing, reasoning and interpretive procedures. For Garfinkel (1967), this is the documentary method of interpretation: the case in 'case records' stands not for an individual case, but as a 'documented representation' of professional and institutional practice. At the same time, Garfinkel (1967: 186–207) captures the situatedness of case notes in the medical setting by talking about '"good" organizational reasons for "bad" clinical records'. He points out that case notes are 'results of self-reporting procedures' and are inevitably selective with regard to the activities of the professionals as they 'actively seek to act in compliance with rules of the clinic's operating procedures that for them and from their point of view are more or less taken for granted as right ways of doing things' (1967: 191). In this sense, case records are an index of professional autonomy and consensus (Barrett 1996, see also Chapter 4 on consensus work in inter-professional case conferences). The consensus aspect gives the documents a stamp of authority, or what Zimmerman sees as the 'plain fact' character of records, and seen as reliable and objective. In this way the records help to turn subjective assessments into objective facts.

With regard to social work, Pithouse (1987) suggests that case records are 'imperfect accounts': not an authentic record of what actually happens in social work practice. Generally speaking, files do not tell the full story. Incompleteness and incoherence is intrinsic to case records, because by definition they are selective for purposes of day-to-day management. Similarly, Hak (1992: 193) points out that 'there is no reality against which psychiatric records can be compared. They can only be studied as a part of psychiatric practice'. To read these entries, says Garfinkel, you must be an insider (very much purpose-driven): 'The crux of the phenomenon lies elsewhere, namely in the ties between records and the social system that services and is serviced by these records.' Pithouse supports his argument by citing comments made by social workers about case notes. He goes on to suggest that the records are 'a negotiable resource', which will be selectively used in the future. This echoes Garfinkel and others about the designated, but so far unknown, audience of case records, including the court and the public inquiry.

In what follows, we will focus on one single case in detail (from which the first file entry above is taken). Case notes involving clients in child welfare share similar linguistic, rhetorical and thematic features. These may include: assessment of family relations; evaluation of at-risk status of children; identification of the perpetrator through character work. In this process social workers often find themselves in the midst of multi-agency collaboration, given the complex nature of institutional intervention. We are also interested in how the case notes construct the client in terms of a cooperative or non-cooperative stance in view of accomplishing a 'preferred' state of family set-up.

Our analytic focus will be on the role which case records play in the organisation of social practice. We address three aspects of categorisation: the categorisation of the client and their family relations; the categorisation of child abuse/neglect as an institutional reality; and the categorisation of social work profession. At the same time, case records show how information is compiled, i.e., when social workers go out to collect information and when information is thrust upon them. This draws our attention to the salience of reported speech (e.g., 'she repeated the information given in her letter'; 'he agreed to ask police to investigate'). This includes self-reporting signalled through the agency of the record-keeper (e.g., 'I asked whether the injury was consistent with the explanation'; 'I said I would be informing police') which reveals the backstage activities being undertaken. Reported speech is of particular significance because it is deployed for strategic purposes: to agree or disagree with a particular state of affairs, to contrast different viewpoints, to arrive at consensus, to attribute agency to participants and to underline the decision-making process etc. (Hall *et al.* 1999a).

There exists a body of literature focusing on the organisational role of case records in social work practice, including social workers' reflective accounts on case records (for a comprehensive overview, see Pithouse 1987 and Prince 1996). Among others, Parton *et al.* (1997) have analysed case records to show how child protection work is multi-faceted and, even where the child is the concern or object, a great deal of family, parenting, etc. assessment is carried out as routine practice.

Social workers in child protection work operate with a variety of checklists and procedures, some formal and explicit others informal and implicit. To what extent do these guide their record keeping? This question reveals a dilemma of practice: do the formal documents constrain or support social workers' assessments and actions? Although discourse scholars have analysed case records in other professional sites (e.g., Barrett 1996; Cicourel 1974; Coulthard 1996; Hak 1992; Jonsson and Linell 1991; Mehan 1983; Pettinari 1988; Ravotas and Berkenkotter 1998; Slembrouck 1992; Zimmerman 1969), social work case records have not been subjected to detailed discourse analysis.

Categorisation of the client and family relations

A key feature of case records is the characterisation of clients, which is otherwise difficult in face-to-face encounters (as indicated in Chapter 5, client charac-terisations will often be less explicit in a home visit). Pithouse (1987: 94) cites the following self-report from a social worker: 'That's how I can best describe the family, of course I don't give that impression when I'm there, who'd want to know they were a reluctant housewife and their house was whiffy . . .' On the one hand, this confession attests to the fact that face-saving strategies may prevent social workers from expressing their 'true' attitudes and feelings when working with clients. The case records then become a means to express 'honest' assessment of clients. On the other hand, this practice is a clear indication of the discrepancy between what might have happened during a visit or in a phone call and what becomes recorded in the file. The reverse scenario is also plausible. Social workers are aware of their limitations when it comes to interpreting other family lives and relations. As Prince (1996) observes, social workers strategically signal their distance from what is recorded in case notes. She provides the account of a psychiatric social worker:

People can describe their families, homes and childhoods and I couldn't write it any better because it sums up in two or three words exactly how they thought or felt. So I use those expressions in inverted commas so others know that it isn't my words.

(Prince 1996: 51)

This also takes care of clients' concern that their words may be interpreted differently – that their own interpretation of events may not be preserved in the official written document.

Generally speaking, clients are usually given more of a voice in case records. There is a sustained attempt at trying to portray the viewpoint of clients and their family. In child welfare cases, the children's voices also have to be heard. There are two dimensions to capturing the client's situation: first, voices of different family members can be selectively recruited as part of client assessment; second, client categorisation has to be achieved through recruiting the voices of other professionals who are involved in the case. Both of these dimensions are oriented towards achieving some kind of consensus.

Although Janice is the main point of contact for the social workers, the welfare of the children remains the priority. There is less characterisation of the father as such, as he is already labelled as the offender. Janice's actions as a mother in this dysfunctional family and also as a client of the social services receive close attention. She is categorised along the following lines: as a non-cooperative client, a deficient parent who fails to protect her children adequately, as an anxious and aggressive person; and as dishonest (an outright moral categorisation). It becomes necessary for the social worker to enlist Janice's cooperation in safeguarding the children by keeping the father away from the house. This necessitates a complex set of activities as Janice does not agree with the social worker that the father is the problem and is adamant that he is neither a threat to her nor to the children. This characterisation of the father by Janice does not coincide with that of the social worker.

The non-cooperative dimension is mainly accomplished through Janice's disagreement with the social services' version of events. She refuses to accept the institutional label attached to the father and blames the social services for the current states of affairs – that the father has been locked up and that the children are being turned against her. Consider the following entries which explicitly mention Janice's disagreement. She is presented as a non-cooperative client. The use of quotation marks in the last entry signals that the expressed views are not endorsed by the social worker (see Prince's point above), and especially in the case of 'he had a right to see his children' we know that the social worker cannot be expected to be in agreement with the mother (as there is a court injunction against the father visiting the home).

Case notes I

(Night duty) said that (mother) felt that (father) was being hard done by and shouldn't be in custody. Angry with Social services. Feels we were making judgements on past violence. Feels strongly that (father) is not guilty – said with a house this big she needs a man around. Feels Social services is turning (child) against her. (19/09)

In my view (mother) was not prepared to accept any role in protecting the children from (father) + indeed felt Social services were to blame for the fact that (father) was locked up + (child) was in (children's home). (18/09)

(Mother) met (father) at his mother's some weeks after the first meeting. He asked to see his children and (mother) invited him to the house. He had been here 'a few times' since then. (Mother) felt 'he had a right to see his children'. I asked if he had threatened her in any way and she said 'no he's not been threatening at all recently'. (18/09 – 3.10pm)

Janice's non-cooperative, disagreeable stance extends to the present concern about the child's broken nose. Although she accepts that the father caused the injury, she insists that it was accidental. She offers an alternative version of the alleged accident:

Case notes 2
(child's) injury was an accident – he was on the bed talking back to [father] who was holding his arm. (Child) bounced awkwardly and his nose broke. (18/09)

There is a caring mother lurking behind this resistant, non-cooperative social work client. This is manifest in her determination not to disrupt the relationship between the father and children; in her insistence to see the children at every possible opportunity when they are in care; and in putting up a continuing resistance to institutional intervention. As we will see, it is this character of Janice which overrides her non-cooperative, aggressive attitude towards social work, when the case comes to court. Even though the father continues to remain a potential offender, this is not enough ground to separate the children from the mother.

Janice is generally portrayed as an anxious mother who is very concerned about the well-being of her children. She justifies the father's presence in terms of children needing him; and she wants someone around in the big house. She upholds the ideals of a happy, integrated family, which includes the father in it. This leniency of the mother in admitting the father into the everyday life sphere of the children can be seen as an expression of 'natural love' (Dingwall *et al.* 1983). But this attitude of Janice remains a matter of concern for the social worker who would like to use this as a basis for taking the children into care. At one stage, Janice is reported as saying 'she wished she was in care'. On two occasions, she is reported as saying 'I would rather kill the children than seeing them in care'. These are double-edged remarks. On the one hand, Janice may be seen as someone who is not able to cope. But on the other hand, she presents a positive image of motherhood: she would rather go into care herself than the children; she would rather kill the children than bear the consequences of them being in care. What comes across in clear terms is that as far as she is concerned the option of children in care is an outright dispreferred option. Her love for the children is starkly juxtaposed to her resistance of social work intervention, as can be seen from the following entry:

Case notes 3

(Mother) phoned v. angry and upset. Didn't want me to visit. I'd taken (child) against his wishes to (children's home). Said she'd kill the kids before we had a chance to take them away from her. I tried to explain that no decisions had been made yet. Felt we needed to talk to her first. She put the phone down still angry + upset. Obviously anxious about what we are going to do. (18/09)

Janice is portrayed as an accomplice, who behaves irresponsibly even when the father is a known risk to the children. This viewpoint also comes across strongly in the interview account (Hall *et al.* 1997b), where the father's actions are clearly marked as 'violent', without the need for cataloguing the details of such violent events. Another dimension of Janice's non-cooperative clienthood concerns her relationship with various professionals. With regard to many of the meetings with fellow professionals, Janice is characterised as anxious and aggressive. Consider the following entries:

Case notes 4

(Health Visitor) said (mother) had come in yesterday to the clinic but only stayed 2 minutes and stormed off – Reason not known. (18/09)

(Mother) then got irate + shouted that she would run off with children or kill them and then herself rather than let them take the 3 younger children. (18/09)

(Mother) left the office accompanied by a woman friend shouting and throwing the fire extinguisher over. (18/09)

(Mother) refused to wait. (19/09)

They (Family Centre) later phoned back to say she'd gone but angry. (19/09)

(Mother) clearly upset when she saw us, she became explosive. (19/09)

Taken together, Janice may be seen as a difficult client to deal with. Her aggressiveness with professional agents contrasts sharply with her anxiousness as a mother who always happens to have the children's well-being at heart. Janice seems to consider the present threat of the father (if that is indeed true) as preferable to a scenario which amounts to children going into care. This axis of non-cooperation finally leads to institutional intervention as is evident from the entry on 19/09 in the case record:

Case notes 5

Discussed with (AM), TL + self. Decision to take children into care today. Reasons:

1) (Mother)'s clear statement that she will not work with Social services in any way.
2) Her view that (father) has right to see children and apparently need to have him around.
3) Dishonesty and the need for (mother) to be honest if there is any chance of working together.

This entry is in stark contrast to the running record style of other entries. It records a meeting, but more than that it lays out a list of justifications, not based on facts but on moral evaluations ('will not work with social services', 'dishonest'). Arguably, it offers a private moment in the case records, in which the social worker displays an amount of exasperation. Note the categoric modality of 'she will not work . . .' and 'any chance', and the irony implied by 'apparently need to have him around'. It is commonplace to provide statements from which inferences can be drawn. This explicit stance is an extreme case formulation with no concessions: it frames social work intervention as undesirable, while acknowledging Janice's competency in dealing with the present situation. Overall, the mother stresses the need for the father–children bonding, even though in the eyes of the social worker, the father is a threat to the children's safety. The only option, from a social work perspective, therefore seems to be to keep the father away from the scene. But if the mother fails to cooperate, and allows the father to see the children behind the social worker's back, as it were, then this counts as a dishonest course of action. It would then follow that the children will need to be taken into care, because no working relationship between the social worker and the mother can be guaranteed.

One critical moment in our case is the event of taking the children to care, which again offers the possibility to categorise Janice as non-cooperative and dishonest. Given the significance of such institutional intervention, we notice entries for 19/09 on an hourly basis. Let us consider in detail the entry for 12 o'clock, which comes across as a thick description of events:

Case notes 6

12.00: AM, team clerk & myself arrived at (mother)'s house at 5.10. We were accompanied by 2 WPCs and a PC. The objective being to take 3 children into care until future plans could be discussed. Decided police should try and get access first, felt this more likely than us. Initially no answer but (mother) finally talked to the WPC through the window. She then let them in. We followed. (Mother) clearly upset when she saw us, she became explosive (see my affidavit sworn on . . .) Decided nothing could be gained trying to talk to (mother). Felt we had no alternative but to take the children as quickly as possible. (Brother) was crying in corner. I picked him up and put him in the car. He calmed v. quickly (again refer to affidavit) as we were passed (park) in the car I made reference to the trip to the zoo this summer – money which was given to (mother) to take them. They said Mum hadn't taken them to the zoo or (park) 'but she had told you (me) that we had'.

This build up suggests that the mother can be potentially difficult to handle. An evaluative tone is present throughout. Apart from displaying the right way of coordinating the act of removing the children from the home, the self-report also shows a number of disruptive events as well as the worker's spontaneous response to these (cf. mother as explosive; 'nothing could be gained trying to talk to mother'). The intensity of details suggests that this is a critical moment for definitive action.

Although children's voices do not appear much in this case record, their voice is strategically recruited in the above entry in order to establish a negative character of Janice. That she has not been honest and truthful is accomplished through reported speech ('they said mum hadn't taken them to the zoo or (park)'). Elsewhere in the record we have glimpses of how the children behaved towards their mother. They are reported as feeling uncomfortable and agitated in Janice's presence, which is sometimes contrasted with their feeling settled in the children's home.

Case notes 7
(Residential social worker) said (child) very quiet + withdrawn

(Mother) was asking if she could visit the next day apparently children went berserk when they saw her v. hyped up + manic (23/09)

Children all over the place while mother was there (24/09)

Within the social work profession, it is widely held that any categorisation of clients can be subjective and value-laden, however much such subjective judgements are routinely backed up with descriptive accounts. It is helpful to compare two entries by two different social workers about the same client (taken from Pithouse 1987: 35–36):

> (Father) has consistently refused to let me enter the house saying he can care for the children quite well 'without you lot'. I explained that I had every right to see the children as they are on supervision. He's an aggressive man with a history of drinking and was under the influence when I spoke to him. He calls me 'love' in a very sarcastic way and is probably worried that I undermine his authority in the house and his image of the 'boss' in the family. I explained that unless he cooperated I would have to go back to court as the supervision order was ineffective . . .

> (Father) sat quietly as his wife talked about (child) and (child), (mother) did most of the talking, about (child)'s truancy and the recent offence. (Father) was evidently upset saying this was the first time (child) had been in trouble. (Mother) asked him to make tea and he returned a little later with biscuits, cups and tray and served the tea. There seemed little of the aggressive father I met some weeks ago. We then discussed the court appearance . . .

Two different pictures about the father's character emerge, but the social worker is quick to point out that the first entry does not amount to failure on the part of the previous social worker. The second entry comes across as positive. In fact the present worker contrasts an earlier depiction of the father as aggressive with the one reported in this instance as 'quiet' and 'upset'. There can be many reasons for such a difference, including of course the presence of the mother who is the main narrator in this meeting. What is striking here is the detailed description of the father's tea making/serving routine which is intended as evidence of why the father cannot be simply characterised as difficult, non-cooperative, aggressive, etc., as suggested by the first entry. The reverse also holds: once a positive assessment of character is made, the descriptive details can be fashioned accordingly. While the first entry carries a threat of a dysfunctional client–social work relationship and consequently a court action, the second offers a sense of optimism and positive outcome.

Returning to our case study, the characterisation of the mother, Janice, as non-cooperative and dishonest assumes more definitiveness as the preparation for the court hearing gathers momentum. With the exception of entries like case notes 5, the entries over two weeks mostly report event work. We have descriptions of the following type: Janice invited father to the house; he had been there 'few times', as well as all those occasions where she stormed out of meetings, became explosive, etc. Several things have been written down, even though one does not know whether these will turn out to be relevant. Such entries record raw material (albeit coloured to an extent) for others to do character work in other places and at other times. The focus on eventness then enables a closer understanding of the character to emerge. In this particular case, the upcoming court case will require a detailed report in which character work will become a central concern. Metaphorically, thick descriptions of events act as a zooming in on the character. Most of the time the behaviour and actions of Janice and other family members are described, without an explicit assessment of character. In other words, categorisations are made available for readers but these are not really undertaken in the case records. The risk the father presents to the children is presumed rather than described in any detail. Several aspects – in rather self-contradicting ways – of the mother's character come out through the accounts provided in the case record: an aggressive but anxious mother, a non-cooperative but determined client. Immediately after the children were taken into care, Janice was reported as admitting 'she was wrong but still didn't understand why we'd taken them' (23/09). This sense of 'being more sinned against than sinning' to some extent anticipates the court decision in favour of children returning home.

Categorisation of child abuse/neglect

Social workers have to work within the institutional categories and types of responses available to them in dealing with particular cases. In the context of physical abuse, they will need to seek actively medical and factual evidence, which necessarily means reporting other professionals' assessment of the case in hand. This is where social work case records resemble medical records, the latter being more about symptoms, diagnosis, treatment at a factual and technical level rather than about social relationships.

Let us return to the case notes we started the chapter with. The incidence and causation of the broken nose needs to be established. We have already seen in the previous section Janice's version, which acknowledges that the father caused it, but puts it down to an accident. This categorisation is consistently denied by the social worker, because accepting it would mean that the father is no longer a risk to the children. The doctor is recruited to provide a factual, scientific categorisation – to make a distinction between the broken nose caused by accident versus the broken nose caused by excessive force. This categorisation is crucial to further action –

whether this is to take children into care and/or to label the father as the perpetrator.

In social work, one would expect clients' words to be represented in their own context – a form of contextualistion which does not distort clients' experience. One reason to use clients' words in case records, according to Prince (1996), is that often social workers fail to understand clients' intended meanings, and so to refrain from imposing their own interpretation. This is particularly significant in the description of actions which may have consequences for institutional categorisation. Leaving clients' words in the case records as they were spoken allows for different inferences to be made in the future. The following account of a social worker concerning sexual abuse, taken from Prince (1996: 52), illustrates this point:

> The teenage girl talked about how her father 'held her'. I couldn't tell if she was describing him embracing her or hitting her, so I wrote down her words as I didn't know what she meant. It was something like he fell onto her – it was ambiguous. She was able to repeat it. I knew it was important but I didn't know what it meant.

When specific client-initiated meanings are not available, categorisation has to be achieved through inter-agency consensus, for it to stand any chance of success when the case goes to court.

Case notes 8

19/09 – 8am: Phoned Police. Informed them of current plans and pre warned them that we possibly were going to need Police help – suggested that we ring back later ask to speak to controller as new shift would be coming on. He informed me that (police doctor) was not prepared to give an opinion as to how the break on (child)'s nose occurred. He has asked a forensic pathologist to give his opinion. (Police) made it clear that information regarding the break was dependent on this otherwise they have no evidence. They are therefore not certain yet as to whether the nose was deliberately (unclear) by (father). Conflicting information from (mother, child & father).

This file entry, while acknowledging conflicting accounts given by different family members, underscores how the police wants to follow its own course via a forensic pathologist in establishing what may have led to the incidence of the broken nose. There is some ambiguity which needs resolving – whether the broken nose is accidental or intentional.

At one point, there is a graphic description of how the father was hysterical when the ambulance came, which included the reaction of the ambulance man: 'Apparently an ambulance man said why is he in such a state why his behaviour is like that if it was an accident?' (23/09). This is an instance of recruiting a third party viewpoint as a way of stressing that there is more than what meets the eye.

Within social work, physical abuse, sexual abuse and neglect are legal categories which are routinely worked up and justified in accounts in order to be able to proceed with care and protection orders. The category of neglect (see Chapters 3 and 7) is more likely to focus on the appropriateness of the care provided for the children, whereas the category of physical abuse is more likely to shift attention to the father as a potential offender. Each category is very likely to be negotiated when applied to individual cases (Hyden and Overlien 2005). Unless a category definition is mutually agreed upon, it is difficult to define the perpetrator.

Professionals who are in positions of institutional authority are 'in a position to give official imprint to versions of reality' (Goffman 1983: 17). Record-keeping in medical, educational and social welfare contexts is one such occasion for giving official imprint to versions of clients' reality (see Mehan (1996) on how the case record becomes institutional reality and indexes decision-making as distributed across participants and across time). In the context of psychiatric institutions, Goffman (1968) points out that case records are an important expression of the institutional mandate. Within the life of a given case, more and more information about those relevant aspects of the professional's definition of the category are included so as to arrive at a fit. This explains obvious omissions made in case notes, for instance, the rare mention of what psychiatric patients are able to do, or their past. 'One of its purposes is to show the ways in which the patient is "sick" and the reasons why it was right to commit him and is right currently to keep him committed; and this is done by extracting from his whole life course a list of those incidents that have or might have had "symptomatic significance"' (1968: 144). In a similar vein, Harré (1985: 179) notes: 'Thus feeling miserable may be described as "displays low affect" to reflect the situational requirements of scientific objectivity embodied in the jargon of psychiatrists'. As Cicourel (1983: 227–228) suggests, 'the physician recodes the patient's often ambiguous, rambling, and somewhat emotional language into fairly abstract categories'. It is interesting that in the medical context, it is a practice of *recoding* – through a process of recontextualisation – rather than simple *recording*. Recontextualisation (Linell and Sarangi 1998) is a routine discoursal activity in many institutional and professional settings where clients' (usually spoken) accounts are transformed into texts in order to fit within the institutional schema (see also Hak 1989). This procedure signals the hierarchical nature of lay-expert knowledge structures and interpretive practices (Sarangi and Slembrouck 1996).

Returning to our case study, it is important to note that although the court decided that 'the children should return home' – which was in effect a recognition of the mother's love for the children – the categorisation of the father as an offender is retained. However, his actions are not considered to be serious abuse, which in effect undermines the social services' version of events. Consider the following entry:

Case notes 9

Judge decided that children should return home. (Child) home at weekends. Plans to continue as before. (Mother) to tell court or Social services if (father) comes back on the scene. Injunction to be reinforced and served on (father). Just before going in we heard (father)'s charges were dropped. Decision for children to go home was based on this knowledge.

To summarise thus far, decision-making is of high priority in social work. Case records provide the grounds on which decisions have to based, e.g., to seek a care order, to go to court, to move the family, to involve other agencies etc. Holland (1999) draws our attention to two types of discourse that social workers deploy in their decision-making practices: discourse of scientific observation and discourse of reflective evaluation. Scientific evidence is what counts when a case goes to court. So, as we have seen, definitions about what constitutes a case of physical abuse and whether the broken nose can be established as caused by force rather than by accident are central to successful intervention.

Categorisation of social work practice

Our final discussion centres on the ways in which case records categorise social work practice, which can include both inter-agency collaboration and clients' perceptions of the role of social workers and the profession itself.

As in other settings, social work case records are organisationally motivated. They are about professional identities and power relations (Pithouse 1987; Prince 1996). They are also accounts of good professional practice. According to Parton *et al.* (1997: 79):

> They (the files) therefore tell us how decisions are accountably arrived at, what is important, appropriate, adequate for practical purposes to say, and not say, to orient to and to leave, to make judgement about and not to judge at all – for organisational (child protection) purposes.

However, there is no denying that the case records consist of self-reports, which combine aspects of ongoingness with retrospective and prospective accounting (Dingwall *et al.* 1983: 80). They are a way of detailed recording for what has happened, current happenings, and future actions and decisions. The retrospective dimension is evident from the following entry:

Case notes 10

Phoned day nursery + informed them of the situation, checked if children had been here since the incident of the bite marks (11–11). They confirmed children in day nursery, were busy at the time. (Mother) refused to wait.

Case records are often referred to in supervision meetings and in case conferences as an accurate record of past actions. The retrospective account also at times includes minute details about the organisation of events, sometimes on an hourly basis, in order to attain completeness/relevance of record keeping.

By contrast, prospective accounting is accomplished at two levels: (1) in terms of what needs to be done (e.g., a checklist of things to do such as to telephone x, to contact y), and (2) to anticipate and prepare for alternative action points:

Case notes 11

Phone call to solicitor to explained situation. If (father) is sent home on bail we will have to think seriously about the risk to the children possibly remove them into care. If he is remanded in custody we can wait until later on in this week to attend High Court (and) make an ex parte application. Agreed to find result of hearing + inform our Area through? (16/09)

More important than the expression of uncertainty about the state of affairs, the entry in case notes 11 signals prospective accounting in that alternative scenarios of intervention are available to the social worker. It also prepares for an account in case a state of affairs materialises. Forward looking scripts entail references to past experiences of similar scenarios, through which the social worker displays competent knowledge. Cicourel has shown that in both legal and medical settings, recording of 'what happened' and the next course of action has to be accomplished within 'the organisational rules and practices for "making sense" of "what happened"' and 'preparing the scene for further inference and action' (1974: 85). According to Prior (2003: 3), 'every document stands in a dual relation to fields of action': the case records are not just repositories of information, they are also an agent in their own right that is open to further action and interpretation.

This combined retrospective-prospective accounting practice at times reveals the active investigative stance of the social worker ('I asked whether the injury was consistent with the explanation'; 'I said I would be informing the police', etc.). This signals the routine nature of professional activities: the right way of doing things and displaying this as such. One interesting aspect of the case notes is the explicit formulation of alternative action scripts for the future and even hypothetical scenarios. In the above entry we see 'if . . . then' constructions. On the one hand, it shows the flexibility and contingent nature of social work intervention. On the other hand, it can be linked to formulation of uncertainty and being prepared for risk management. In this sense case records are part of reflexive accounting, which is self-critical but also a display of 'doing all the right actions'. As Garfinkel (1967) points out, there are constraints of a general nature on self-reporting in the institutional context mainly because of the uncertainties about how an entry will be interpreted in the future. Moreover, the report is now produced for a particular audience and for a specific purpose, although what constitutes the audience and the purpose will vary across contexts and across time.

The complexity of social work cases, especially with child welfare, requires inter-professional collaboration. Case records give accounts of such collaboration work, including aspects of disagreement and non-cooperation. The multiple perspective is used for consensual purposes to show agreement in decision-making:

Case notes 12

SW & TL discussed case with Senior Manager, Agreed:

1. Phone her solicitor + inform her of invitation to visit her at home.

2. Check with (legal department) to confirm Registrar informed of (child)'s injury.

3. Home visit to be made to (mother) to ask her a) what was her opinion of cause of

(child)'s injury. b) what is her explanation as to (father's) presence into house. c) given (mother)'s lack of openness + honest over cooperation with SW, i.e. not informing SSD of (father)'s visit to the house, what is the realistic prospect of social work role continuing to provide protection to the children. (18/09 – 12.15)

In the case record we have explicit statements about the relationship between the client and social work.

Case notes 13

I asked (mother) what future she saw in working with SSD. She said she couldn't talk to (SW) and didn't want anymore 'mealy mouthed' social workers. Social services just bribed her with carpets, washing machines, etc.

Here social work is characterised as 'mealy mouthed', 'bribing' her into consensus and not recognising the need for children to have access to father, etc. In other words, we get a sense of a dysfunctional relationship between the family and the social work profession, giving rise to two competing versions of events.

When the case goes to court, it is the mother's version that triumphs. In the interview account (Hall *et al.* 1997b), the social worker summarises: 'we went back to court for a fuller hearing . . . Janice was able to put her side of the story and we put our side of the story and the judge decided that the children should go back home'. What we have here is a clear acknowledgement that case records do not necessarily represent the client's side of the story, despite the fact that client voices are reported in abundance throughout the record.

As we have seen, the entries are particularly detailed at strategic moments. This means that one could look at the intensity of entries and identify what constitutes a strategic moment in professional work. One reason behind such detailed reporting may be the display of professional competency. But looked at from a different angle, tremendous detail in case records may support or undermine the image of competent social work. This is particularly so when recorded details are not about strategic moments (e.g., 'sister extremely active running in + out of doctor's consulting room . . . Finally (RSW) brought her a cup of tea'). Such details may be part of a display of competent observation, yet its relevance can be put to question. It is possible to argue that there is a tension between minute observation and accurate record-keeping on the one hand, and its prospective relevance on the other hand. One possible reason for entering such details may be the uncertainties surrounding future scenarios and possible decisions. There is something about certain situations of child abuse where social workers take down 'everything', working with a notion of completeness/faithfulness. As Kagle (1993) puts it: 'Like physicians who have learned to practise defensive medicine, social workers have learned to practise and record defensively'. According to Walker, Shemmings and Cleaver (2005), 'under recording' can also serve a defensive purpose in a climate of increasing professional accountability.

Pithouse (1987) dwells on the reflective dimension of the case record – e.g., how it is used for supervision and protection purposes, especially when it concerns a novice professional whose practices are not directly observable. For novices, case records then become a form of 'legitimate peripheral participation' in Lave and Wenger's (1991) terms. Case records, according to Goffman (1968), can also contribute towards colleagues learning about a patient or a criminal. But, as we have seen, in the case of social work fellow professionals may express cynicism and treat previous entries with caution: 'You try not to let the file colour you, assessments change' (Pithouse 1987: 34). Social work case records are necessarily judgemental, so this is given as a reason for not reading them in detail. The cynicism is best expressed in the following example taken from Pithouse (1987: 38):

> Social worker to team leader and the researcher: Look! (holding manila file) I've had this case and I've been able to do nothing with them (clients) but I've made it <u>look</u> (her emphasis) dynamic (laughs). Well you've got to give some impression even if you can't do much – I dress it up with long words to fill the gaps, you see nothing has happened, but you have to write something . . .

This 'burden of recording' is the protecting dimension as far as social work is concerned. However imperfect, case records also serve a more practical purpose in professional settings. Rather than becoming documents in their own right, they become prompts for the production of formal assessment reports, especially in therapeutic settings (Hak 1992; Ravotas and Berkenkotter 1998). Barrett (1996) rightly shows how case notes can also influence future activities. Doctors routinely consult previously recorded case notes in an ongoing consultation. In the context of social work, case records form a part of the proceedings of case conferences and also as part of the court proceedings. In the case we have been analysing, explicit entries are made to avoid case conferences on grounds of urgency as well as when a case conference is to be called.

Conclusion

Case notes are both public and private arenas of social work. There is no doubt that record keeping is a particular professional site where professional competencies and organisational procedures can be analysed. In citing Margolin (1997) and Tice (1998), Floersch (2004: 164) provides a compelling account of how case records allow researchers to make knowledge claims of the following kind: '(1) social workers non-reflexively controlled clients by keeping close watch and writing detailed case records; and, (2) case records functioned to invent and reproduce social work as a profession'.

Hayes and Devaney (2004) go to the extent of expressing concerns about increasing regulations in accessing case records for research purposes. In a number of areas like institutional audit, professional supervision, etc. case notes are used to assess professional practice. Our interest here has been with understanding case notes as yet another site for categorising the client and displaying the practices of social workers.

In addition to difficulties about accessing of case records, there is also the problem of interpreting case records. In the context of medical practice, Garfinkel (1967) alerts us to the fact that case records defy easy interpretation, especially from an outsider perspective. It is important to recognise that case records need to be interpreted in terms of their intended audience, which are often fellow professionals (see Garfinkel's distinction between actuarial and contractual readings of case documents). He suggests that the interpretation of such records is indeterminate from the perspective of the writer, or what he terms as the 'elected scheme of interpretation'. 'The present circumstances of the reader in deciding their appropriate present use' overrides 'the circumstances that accompanied the original writing' (1967: 202). This may partly explain why fellow social work professionals can raise doubts about previous observations made in a given case record. The information contained in the case notes is for 'future but unknown purposes'. This is the occasionality dimension of interpretation. In the context of social work, this could be other members (as in the case conference when decisions about appropriate intervention have to be made) or the legal system when a case goes to court or becomes the subject of public inquiry. This is unpredictable and this is what makes such record-keeping difficult.

The significance of case records with regard to the construction of professional practice is, however, underscored by the fact that social historians analyse case records to understand the organisation of the social work profession. In this sense, they are like ethnographic fieldnotes, grounded in the everyday realities of people. If case conferences and supervision meetings with team leaders are oral accounts about clients ('telling the case', to use Pithouse's term), then case records are written accounts about clients which amount to 'writing the case'. In both ways the 'invisible trade' of social work is made visible. While some may detect the paradox that what is made visible does not reflect what goes on in 'real' practice, we prefer to argue that it involves translation from one arena of practice to another. Note the significance which the barrister in a public inquiry gives to case notes, treating them as 'real practice'. Case notes remain open to inferences and interpretations in selective ways at another time, as we have seen with our case study when the case goes to court.

It is this open nature of case records – different interpretations are possible – which has recently come under attack. As Walker, Shemmings and Cleaver (2005) point out, the sheer size of the record and its narrative, discursive style can pose problems for locating key information, with the risk of important information being overlooked. A further – and more important – concern is what does not get recorded. In the wake of the publication of the Victoria Climbié Inquiry Report (Laming 2003), all agencies involved have come under criticism for missing out relevant details and for the failure to bring together pivotal assessments (Rustin 2005).

Already case notes are being transformed. As electronic record-keeping becomes a norm (also in the case of medical case records), there is now a call for greater regulation and governance on how records are kept. Call for such a change in recording practice is in line with greater accountability on the part of professionals. However, standardised structured responses run the risk of professionals simply recycling institutional categories, that is, getting into the practice of recording what institutional agencies want to hear, rather than capturing the complexity of events and characters as we have seen in our case study.

In the context of social work, the suggested changes to format, i.e., electronic case records, go beyond a simple change of medium. It will inevitably influence content, and thus social work practice. For instance, how will such record-keeping affect the remit of case conference? The case of integrated electronic records is very much made along the lines of sharing of information and moving away from the provisional nature of paper records (Hardstone *et al.* 2004). Looking at our case study, it is clear how many phone calls are made (see for instance the entry on 19/09), which result in unending reporting of other voices. With an electronic system, other professionals can easily enter their own accounts. Rather than the onus being on the social worker to justify his/her actions to fellow colleagues and the higher management within social services, social work practice may become more other-oriented.

To what extent will the 'personal' orientations of social work professional practice, as epitomised in case records, become a contested domain in light of the new developments towards electronic record-keeping and record sharing across agencies? Will social workers be allowed a space in which they can let off steam, as for instance was the case in case notes 5. Garfinkel (1967) warns about the difficulties associated with changes in recording practice because this is intricately tied up with professional ethos. In addition, the legal framework – as embodied in the Access to Personal Files Act (1987) and the more recent Freedom of Information Act (2005) – is bound to have implications for how case records are maintained, utilised and how access to them is managed.

7 Parents' accounts of social work

71 CL: [. . .] which I must admit I did have a drink (.) but then again I wasn't just drunk I was just absolutely (.) totally shattered (3) and I had no one else to help me (2) and it's a difficult situation when your boyfriend walks out on ya (.) he don't care the baby's screaming and hollering (4) and you don't dare ring him (.)

72 INT: so

73 CL: this is a sob-story isn't it (laughs)

74 INT: no no no I mean (.) I can understand it must have been very frightening

75 CL: frightening (.) it was bloody awful (.)

In the extract above, we hear a lone mother, Hilary [CL], describe the night she rang social services for help. It takes only a few seconds to learn about the complexities of differentiated role identities: this narrative is not only about a mother caring for a child and a parent having to cope; it is just as much about an individual facing adult life in a network of relationships ('I must admit I did have a drink' and 'I had no one else to help me'). Note in particular how the parenting dimension is constructed as dependent on these relationships ('and it's a difficult situation when your boyfriend walks out on ya . . . he don't care the baby's screaming and hollering . . . and you don't dare ring him . . .').

In the extract above, the mother also dismisses the adequacy of the interviewer's characterisation of the experience of the removal of the child as 'very frightening'. She responds: 'frightening . it was bloody awful'. There is something unusual about this reflexive comment: it comments on the interview situation itself. In turning our attention to the voice of the mother, we are alerted to alternative forms of troubles-telling. For her, the story is personal and deeply emotional: it describes a feeling of being devastated, of feeling at a loss and angry, of lost credibility and not knowing for sure what exactly is going on. The comment 'this is a sob-story isn't it?' frames the categorisation for the interviewer without undermining its absolute nature. It underlines the interactive nature of the telling: even the description of deeply felt emotions happens in response to the context of the telling. There is a significant body of research on parental perspectives on child welfare, especially with a consumer orientation (for example, Cleaver and Freeman 1995; Packman and Hall 1997; Spratt and Callan 2004; Tunstill and Aldgate 2000); however, little of this research acknowledges the context in which such perspectives are articulated. It is assumed that the data gathered is a more or less accurate reflection of what the client thinks about social work intervention. The approach to interview data discussed in Chapter 3 acknowledges the interactive nature of the research task and its events (Slembrouck 2004). However, as the quotation shows, the interviewee displays her awareness that she is producing a formulation of events which can be heard as a 'sob-story', that is, as being of a type and perhaps not necessarily a description of facts and hard-and-fast categories, that states of affairs can be described but their significance is amenable to different attributions of import.

In a number of ways the present chapter offers a mirror image of Chapter 3 which focuses on social workers' narrative constructions of client categories as part of presenting their work as professional, as accountable and as competently handling crisis and institutional intervention. The chapter here therefore raises the question of an alternative account, one which centres on the client's experiences during the height of crisis and after the child had been removed (the visits at the foster home, the case conferences, the counselling and other steps that need to be taken to get the child to return home). The account analysed in this chapter may thus give a few indications as to how the mother challenges the applied categories of the professional and how she resists blame, by accounting for her own behaviour during the period of intervention.

Hilary's immediate audience is the researcher/interviewer. Her child, Michael, was voluntarily admitted into foster care the morning after she had contacted social services for help the night before and a first visit has been made to the house. Later, it transpires that the grandparents and others had already been in contact with social services about the mother's situation. At the time of the interview, the child is still in care. Note, finally, that the account does not develop as a straightforward narrative in the sense of one extended, uninterrupted turn. Instead, a particular causal chronology can be seen to develop implicitly as a narrative emerges in the interactional dynamics of the interviewer's successive questions and the client's responses to these.

The analysis will concentrate on three themes: the client's expectations when inviting an intervention, her responses to social workers' interpretations and her challenge and qualification of the diagnostic categories. In the concluding discussion of implications for practice we will briefly introduce a second case, in which the parents dispute the justification of a particular intervention. What are the consequences of adopting a stance which the client experiences as accumulative criticism and unilateral blaming? Should the social worker try to look for more constructive dialogue or is the undermining of the parent's moral character a requirement before taking a child into care?

Expectations – (5-second pause) 'I didn't know what to make of them to tell you the truth'

Hilary had not had previous contact with social services. In this section, we will discuss her reactions to that initial contact. The account provides various instances where the client expresses surprise at the actions and assessments of the social workers. Already in the first few minutes of the interview (see extract 1 below), when asked if things could have been handled differently, we hear the client's challenge to the inevitable causality between her 'not coping' and the decision to remove the child. On the face of it, the decision is made instantly: the mother gave a signal for help; instead of providing that help, her life was turned upside down even further.

Interview 1 – extract 1

86 INT: oh yeah (laughter) at that point (.) I mean obviously you were very distressed and very confused but (2) what do you think could have been done . how could the thing . could or should things have been done differently (.)

87 CL: erm (.) I think they could have given me (.) I suppose obviously they could have given me time overnight (.) but they could have not done it as fast as what they did (.) like whip him out straight away (.) they could have given me time to settle down . and settle help everything that was going wrong in my life

88 INT: yeah

89 CL: instead of just whipping him away (.) obviously they were concerned which I agree with them they were concerned about his health his chest infection and everything (.) so they were concerned about him which is only natural and I was concerned about him as well . that's why I kept calling out the doctor at night and everything (5) I didn't know what to make of them to tell you the truth

90 INT: okay erm (.) so they took him away you signed the papers (.) did

91 CL: he's in voluntary care

92 INT: yeah

93 CL: it's voluntary not (.) they didn't actually take him I mean they took him as in voluntary.

94 INT: yeah

95 CL: and they always stressed that he is in voluntary care

96 INT: did they make that clear to you at the time

97 CL: no (.) not at the time the (.) person (.) who took him away in the morning didn't actually make it clear unless it was me (.) because I was in such a distressed state at the time because he was being taken away that I didn't actually take it in that he was making clear (.) but they didn't actually give me . I was told that I was going to get a plan thing for him which I didn't get (3) so I thought they knew what they were doing . they're the (.) they're the higher-ups (.) I'm just me I'm just the baby's mother

In the extract transcribed above, the mother responds affirmatively to the interviewer's first question: an alternative cause of action could/should have been available. It is made available in a three-item list (turn 87): 'they could have given me time overnight . . . but they could have not done it as fast as what they did . . . like whip him out straight away . . . they could have given me time . . . to settle down . . . and settle help everything that was going wrong in my life'. Yet, at the same time, a formulation is developed in which the client concedes that the intervention was based on a necessary and justifiable concern: 'obviously they were concerned which I agree with . . . which is only natural'. However, this was a concern which the professionals should have recognised as shared by the mother, and this they didn't. She adds immediately (turn 89): 'and I was concerned about him as well . that's why I kept calling out the doctor at night and everything'. 'Everything that was going wrong in my life' in the client's first turn hints at a set of circumstances invoked. These are later specified as quoted in the preliminary extract at the beginning of the chapter: she wasn't coping, the boyfriend had walked out on her and was not prepared to look after the child, no one was offering any help, etc. The client's concession that the situation had become serious is underscored towards the end of the extract when she admits that she may not have 'taken in' at the time of the intervention that her case counted as 'voluntary care'[1] or that this was being made clear to her (turn 97). The mother was taken by surprise and admits she was in such a state where she may no longer have been able to assess fully what exactly was going on during the intervention. This concession can be read as either underlining the need for the intervention (if the mother was in such a state, how can she be expected to look after her child adequately) and/or as criticising its drastic nature, unjustifiably quick, and characterised by a lack of communicative support.

While the interviewer appears to be interested in the legal notion of whether or not the status of 'voluntary care' was explained adequately ('and did they make that clear to you at the time?', turn 96), the mother downplays any criticism. And, even though she does not want to take full responsibility for the events leading up to the reception into care and questions the justifiability of the drastic decision taken by social services, she also makes clear that she has in fact taken (and is still taking) part of the blame. One could use the term 'event-led self-blaming' here, accomplished through references to the circumstances of her life and institutional decision-making, but in both cases implying a redemption of the client's moral worth and character vis-à-vis the interviewer. The statement, 'I didn't know what to make of them to tell you the truth', in turn 89, is preceded by an unusually long pause. It is an evaluative formulation which sums up her defeated expectations.

The institutional representatives failed to read her alarm signals the way she had intended them to be read. The unexpectedness of the child's removal ('I thought they might help' in the extract immediately below) is explained partly by invoking a mismatch in perceptions:

Interview 1 – extract 2

44 INT: no (.) what did you think they might

45 CL: I thought they might help because I've got a booklet over there actually which I've put picked up in their place which says that they can help you by having someone in during the day to (.) lessen the burden on you (2)

46 INT   what sort of thing were you thinking of there

47 CL   (3) erm (.) to tell you the truth I didn't really know exactly what I was thinking (.) I was thinking they might help me in a more in a different way than they would (.) no way did I think they would whisk my child off me

[. . .]

350 INT: sure it does (.) but is there any particular thing that erm (.) that parents (.) if you. well is there anything you'd have liked someone had said to you before all this

351 CL: make sure you can get a social worker that you can trust

352 INT: yeah (2)

353 CL: and make sure you know exactly what you are doing before you get in contact with them

The client had expected a different course of action, but as she realises now she had misconstrued some of the information provided by the institution itself. Institutional literacy surfaces again towards the end of the interview when the talk returns to the topic of information supply. Asked what she wished she would have known beforehand, the client responds with two pieces of advice to other parents.

Although largely articulated negatively as absent from this particular case (these social workers could not be 'trusted' and therefore it is important to 'know exactly what you are doing before you get in contact with them'), the two pieces of advice can equally be read as a characterisation of how to maintain control over social work intervention – either you can trust the social worker to act in your best interest or try to manage the nature of the intervention. 'Trust' appears here as a very complex category. It involves both the acceptance of the authority and professional competence of social workers as well as the insistence that they will not act against the client. Note in particular how the latter is linked explicitly to institutional literacy. 'Trust' here means that institutional representatives should ensure that the client possesses knowledge of the extent and consequences of any initiated courses of action and that readings of a situation will not result in a mismatch (for instance, the way in which the signing of papers is taken to mean an understanding of the nature of 'voluntary care' in extract 1). The double-advice echoes the client's final turn in extract 1 above. 'They're the higher-ups (.) I'm just me I'm just the baby's mother' not only highlights a power asymmetry, it also brings out the professionals' responsibilities and accountability towards the client. Is this to be heard mainly as an accusation or, does it, conversely, mostly count as a display that the client trusts the professional to know best?

What we have seen in these extracts is the difficulty of the client to understand the actions of the professionals, their claims to authority and where she fits into these practices. She agreed there was a problem, but she has difficulties with the extreme nature of the response. Here, the nature of client participation is in a state of flux.

Performing the client/mother role – 'she was upset with me because I didn't do the usual thing'

Clients, like professionals, do work which displays the complexity of the situation in which they find themselves. Just as the social worker in Chapter 3 had difficulties with a straightforward and simple categorisation as 'child sex offender' or 'failure to thrive', this client experiences difficulty displaying what sort of mother she was when the child was taken away.

Interview I – extract 3

76 INT: so what (.) after that first meeting what what sort of contact what what were what were they saying to you at that stage did they (.)

77 CL: erm (2) I can't remember exactly what happened on the Thursday night because I was so distressed about (.) Michael and worried about him and everything (.) and they came back on the Friday morning . and they came in here (.) gave me a few forms to sign (.) and I said are you taking my baby away from me and they said yes we are (.) and I said why (.) they said because he hasn't been eating properly and (2) and I'd explained to them he had a chest infection problem and wasn't eating properly anyway (.) and they said they were going to take him away and I said what right now and they said yes pack his bags type of thing . and I thought shock horror (unclear) and they were using the phone to phone up people to get him to go round the foster place (.) and I was sitting in total shock I thought I've got no one here with me . I was I was sitting on that chair there thinking there's these two people who've taken my child away from me and I can't do nothing to fight against it (5) and I was so upset and then (.) one of them said to me (.) couple of days later (.) when I got him back for a while (.) she was upset with me because I didn't cry or do do the usual thing when a mother has her baby taken away from her (.) and I said to her what do you expect me to do get angry with you . there's no point in getting angry because if I got angry it would have made it even worse (3) no I was in shock . if you're in shock you don't get angry . sometimes people do . they're angry they get in shock and sometimes they don't (.) I didn't I was just totally (.) devastated I suppose

The extract offers a description of her mental state. The client describes herself as 'distressed', 'worried', and 'in (total) shock', and yet she is criticised by professionals for a lack of public emotional display. The first part of the turn contains a series of little events invested with intense emotions. She recalls procedural detail and makes use of reconstructed dialogue to lend authenticity to the stressful experience. The listener is not only made aware of her intense emotions, he is brought into the picture: 'I was sitting on that chair there'. This is then contrasted with the expectations of the social workers. The social worker's identification that the child was not eating is contrasted with an explanation in terms of a chest infection. There is also the received wisdom that mothers will cry or protest angrily when their baby is taken away from them (but she didn't and this upset one of the social workers): 'if you're in shock you don't get angry . sometimes people do . they're angry they get in shock and sometimes they don't (.) I didn't I was just totally (.) devastated I suppose'. The client and social workers place interpretations on the same set of events, which can become consequential as more serious actions are raised. In a detailed comparison of subsequent reports of client–professional interaction in a child protection case, Urek (2004: 12) notes how the client's 'words, her points of view, her voice were only used for the purpose of confirming the statements of others, they can only support other voices'.

Hilary's account details quite a few instances where she responds to assumptions which she believes institutional workers to hold about 'what mothers do' and 'how good clients behave'. In each case, the comparison of the self with these assumptions is reported to speak against the client's case. As we move on in the sequence of narrated events, there is the mother's report that she felt inhibited when she was visiting Michael at the foster parents' home (in the extract immediately below), as well as her being intimidated during the case conference (our next extract after this).

Interview I – extract 4

140 INT: (foster parent) that's right yeah did did she . discuss with you what what you would do when you went there or or or was it just

141 CL: it was all discussed what we would do and everything . but I was still unsure I'm very (.) when I go round to someone else's house I feel very (2) sort of you don't like to sit in someone else's house and (.) sort of move around in someone else's house (.) it's not your own house is it

142 INT: n- (overlapping)

143 CL: you feel sort of (.) as though you're intruding in someone else's house (.) even though she made me feel (.) very welcome and everything (.) it still wasn't my own house to walk about in

144 INT: right (3) so this sort of started from the first day and then presumably there was a meeting fairly soon was there (.) usually there is or should be

The interviewer is querying the extent to which the mother was visiting the foster home and what the purpose was ('what you would do when you went there'). The context here is that of being assessed while at the foster parents' house. The client outlines the circumstances which, despite the friendliness and welcoming gestures of the foster parents, stopped her from displaying motherhood in the way she knows herself to be capable of. As with the inability to show emotion, the client appears unable to conform to the requirements of the social workers, i.e., continued care for the child. Instead, she is displaying a legitimate characterisation of the self as a reasonable person (despite the consequences).

A similar question of interpretative mismatch surrounds the client's account of her participation in the first case conference. She walked out. What kind of client did that make her in the eyes of the professionals present there? In this case conference, she was supported by a volunteer!

Interview I – extract 5

228 INT: and and did (the volunteer) help you put over your point of view in any way or

229 CL: no actually she she put it over for me

230 INT: ah

231 CL: she stuck up for me . coz I couldn't put it over myself because I felt (2) intimidated by the social services (.)

232 INT: certainly in some people talked about that that at meetings like that and others that there the parents should always have somebody who who's just there to do that . to help parents put their point of view forward (.) and that should

always be the case (.) okay so that was the first meeting (.) at the end of that meeting what sort of s- were any sort of decisions made about what should or shouldn't happen next (.)

233 CL: well I definitely wasn't going to get Michael back (.) I must admit I did walk out on that first meeting coz I cried . I got upset and walked out as there were too many people (.) what I felt was against me

234 INT: yeah

235 CL: I got pretty upset (.) so I walked out . I didn't mean to walk out but I thought I'm not going to cry in front of people I'm going to go outside and have a good cry

236 INT: oh right oh ok ok

The normative point of view is that in a case conference clients are given a space to speak and they may need some assistance in this. Hilary, however, rejects any suggestion that she can put over her point of view in such a setting and allows the volunteer to do this for her: 'I felt intimidated by the social services' (turn 231). It is not clear whether it is the social work meeting or her general orientation to the social work intervention which poses the problem. Next, the interviewer asks about the outcomes of the meeting. Again, in response, the client turns to the detail of her emotional state (she got upset, she walked out, 'too many people what I felt was against me', turn 233).

Extracts 3 to 5 in various ways raise the question of discrepancies between client and social worker interpretations of client motives and behaviours: at the time when the child was being removed, during the first case conference and again during access at the foster parent's house. The client's primary challenge reads that the social workers may not have been getting the full picture of her behaviours and intentions, because they were not understanding the sort of person she was (she keeps her feelings to herself, she doesn't feel happy in other people's houses, she can't express herself in meetings). These are aspects of her personality and it is inappropriate for them to be seen as features of her mothering capacities. Others in similar circumstances may well respond differently.

Challenging and qualifying the diagnostic categories – 'caring but not coping'

This is an account of a mother which is organised around explaining the circumstances of the intervention and in which the client is both handling blame and challenging implications of problematic parenting. For instance, above we have already hinted at how the failure to perceive the concern about Michael as shared between the mother and the social services is argued to have set in motion a procedure which was unjustifiably drastic. In previous work (Slembrouck and Hall 2003), we have identified a feature in which parents address the problem of managing the criticisms of social workers by accepting that they are facing problems (they are not coping) but maintaining their love for their children (they care). In this way, they are able to preserve their moral integrity. Hilary's account provides another example of this, although it is different in that the rhetorical figure is presented here in direct response to the categories recommended by the case conference.

A first occurrence is where the client stresses how, while she may not have been coping, she definitely did care, as she initiated a request for help and she knew she wasn't coping. While there was unanimity between the mother and the social services, the moral assessments that followed from that were different:

Interview 1 – extract 6

61 CL: and they came in and they (2) they were watching me (2) obviously they thought I couldn't cope with Michael which I (.) I knew I couldn't anyway because that's what I asked for help in the first place

A much clearer separation of the 'caring mother' from the person who 'fails to cope' occurs when Hilary directly addresses the categories of child protection, in particular the categories of 'child neglect' and 'child abuse'. The case conference was going to register her as 'likely to abuse her child', a category which she resisted vehemently then and now.

Interview 1 – extract 7

99 CL: mm that's what they said to me that they'd have to go to court (.) and I went to my solicitor . the solicitor didn't see the thing . the first point (.) why he should be kept away from me (2) cos I hadn't really done anything wrong . and when I went to the case conference thing (.) they were going to put down a thing that he was likely to be abused and I went absolutely mad at that because there was no way I'd abuse my son . at all (4) not at all he was neglected . as they put it down he was neglected

100 INT: mmm

101 CL: which he wasn't intentionally neglected . it was because I wasn't feeling too well myself it wasn't (.) what what I always understand as neglection is someone like locking a child away in a bedroom shutting the door and just forgetting about them . whereas I was trying to feed him (.) I was trying to do everything that was right for him . perhaps I was trying too hard (.) because like being a first time mother (.) you try a bit too hard and you're not exactly sure what to do

102 INT: yeah

103 CL: and that's why you ask people for help and then people sometimes when you ask them for help they over-help you . you're not doing this right you're not doing that right (.) do this do that we used to do this we used to do that (.) when you ask for too much help you get overwhelmed you know (4) but I never did nothing wrong with my son (.) and that's what I can't understand (.) I didn't intentionally do anything wrong . and it makes me feel bad now . it's making me feel worse and worse because he's kept away from me for so long (.) and I never did anything wrong (.) I mean I'd understand if I'd (.) coshed him around the head or something like the neighbours complained that he was

crying (.) and when . I saw these counsellor people they said it's understandable that a baby'll cry . that is what a baby does because a baby can't talk . so it cries so of course the neigh the neighbours I used to ask them and that really bugs me about the neighbours I used to say to them can you hear Michael crying (.) and they said no we never hear him crying (.) he's a lovely baby and all things like that and the next thing I know it's written in one of the reports at the (.) social thing (.) that they'd phoned up and said that the baby was crying all the time (.) and I thought to myself what two-faced people there are around here (2) and you can't help a baby crying (.) it's like a dog . you can't help a dog barking can ya (.)

104 INT: just uh
105 CL: sounds awful doesn't it (laughter)
106 INT: no no
107 CL: sounds awful
108 INT: well it sounds yeah it sounds very difficult
109 CL: I mean if a baby cries a baby cries (.) you can't . stop a baby from crying . I mean you don't intentionally leave a baby (.) on the floor crying

Hilary refuses to accept the category of 'likely to abuse' and does so by elaborating a number of arguments in great detail. She particularises the categories of 'abuse' and 'neglect' by offering her own definition with examples, with attendant claims which normalise her child's behaviour: 'there was no way I'd abuse my son' (turn 99) and 'he wasn't intentionally neglected . it was because I wasn't feeling too well myself' (turn 101). Intentional neglect is 'like locking a child away in a bedroom shutting the door and just forgetting about them . whereas I was trying to feed him (.) I was trying to do everything that was right for him. And again further down (turn 103): 'I didn't intentionally do anything wrong . and it makes me feel bad now . it's making me feel worse and worse because he's kept away from me for so long (.) and I never did anything wrong (.) I mean I'd understand if I'd (.) coshed him around the head'. There is the questionable nature of so-called 'evidence/ actions' from neighbours, relatives, etc. who had contacted the social services before she called for help (turn 103). Although Hilary is casting herself as a voluntary client, the social workers were already on to her. The authority of professional voices is invoked in support of her analysis (turn 103): 'I saw these counsellor people they said it's understandable that a baby'll cry . that is what a baby does because a baby can't talk'. Finally, there is the appeal to the experience of being a first time mother ('you try a bit too hard and you're not exactly sure what to do', turn 101). So while the client admits to the category of 'neglect' (expressing her relief that this is not seen as 'abuse'), her 'not coping' is differentiated from 'intentional neglect' ('I was trying to do everything that was right for him', turn 101). The definition of 'neglect' which she offers is an event-definition which can be evidenced (cf. 'locking a child away in a bedroom [. . .] and just forgetting about them', turn 101, and further down 'cosh him around the head or something', turn 103). For social workers, however, 'neglect' is located in the effect on the child rather than the intentions of the parents.

Hilary's line is that she is a caring mother who has made a few mistakes and these make her feel very bad. She confesses to the mistakes she made, while insisting that a larger picture should be looked at which recognises both her 'not coping' and 'caring', instead of just the mistakes which led to a very quick decision to remove the child. As far as she is concerned, the social workers messed her around. However, from a social work point of view, the child's well-being will be the primary concern. For them, it is the situation here and now which, in the interest of the child, requires an intervention: mitigating circumstances do not exonerate parents from being responsible for the present situation as inviting a particular concern. Therefore, the role of the parent is important but secondary, as ultimately the intervention is about the child. An assessment of the parent's cooperation in a procedure, their capabilities, skills, alignment with analysis and their moral character, etc. are secondary and instrumental as guarantees sought for the well-being of the protected child.

Powerlessness of the client when faced with scrutiny by the social services

Clients will tend to see these things differently. While Hilary may say little about the child, she does see herself as under scrutiny from the social worker's point of view; her own parenting or moral character having been discredited. Aren't parents always likely to interpret institutional decisions to place a child as a challenge to their own moral character? In the case of adolescents/teenagers they may not necessarily do so (parents may hold their children responsible – esp. when an institutional intervention follows a teenager's transgression of rules – truancy, petty crime, etc. – and 'no longer coping' becomes 'no longer being able to contain/control' – Slembrouck 2003). In contrast, in the case of small infants, a removal of the child will almost necessarily be read by parents as a defamation of their moral character, a point which the mother is aware of. This is detailed in the following extract where she talks about the initial visit by two social workers, immediately after she had rung social services:

Interview I – extract 8

55 CL: I phoned up Thursday (4) actually I can't remember exactly what happened (.) cos it was such a (.) sort of fast acting thing . such a (8) cos I was feeling so (.) down and whatever and probably cos couldn't contact anyone else I turned to them (2) and they came and they saw me the state I was in

56 INT: they actually came round did they

57 CL: yeah (.) two came round (2) and they saw that I wasn't coping very well with Michael (.) which (.) I tried to explain to people that I wasn't coping with Michael it's a very difficult thing to explain to people that you're not coping with a baby very well

The final utterance in the second turn sums this up: 'it's a very difficult thing to explain to people that you're not coping with a baby very well'. The extract also shows the way events quickly spin out of control – 'a sort of fast acting thing'.

In a wider sense, this raises another set of problems related to the 'presentation of the self': when particular institutional sequences are read by clients in accusatory terms, they face a double problem: a rebuttal will be heard as the primary – and in some cases, the only – course of action available. However, some parents will feel even inhibited to defend, as the mother-client reports in this particular case:

Interview 1 – extract 9

177 CL: there were supposed to be eight I think they told me that there were supposed to be (2) eight people there someone told me I can't remember who told me there was supposed to be eight people there and there ended up being twenty people . I walked into the room (.) and I was nervous as it was . because obviously you're going into something that's like like a judge and jury on you . and you walk in and I looked at all these people and I thought (.) right there . and I thought to myself (.) I've got to sit here in front of all these people being judged . and I sat there like a (.) like that waiting to see what they were judging me on (.) like police people . solicitors . people from the social . Whatever (.) my mum my dad (.) boyfriend solicitors (.)

178 INT: did you know what everyone was . not you kn- (overlapping)

179 CL: well everyone introduced themselves like they do . they all go round the table but you don't (.) but can't really take it all in because there are so many people there and they're all going . hello my name is

180 INT: mm

181 CL: whatever and then you have to introduce yourself . but when you you feel like you're on trial (.) you don't really take it in what's going on around you you sort of (.) they say my name is whatever (.) you have to sort of . you have to acknowledge them but you don't really take it in (.) especially when you're sitting by the door (.) with your coat on your arm

182 INT: (laughter)

183 CL: I'm I'm just the mother . I'm just the baby's mother (.) and then Michael was sitting in the corner there . he was like down there in the corner (.) and all I was taking notice of really was I was half listening to them half watching him because I hadn't seen him in the morning I mean he was my child and I just wanted to pick him up and play with him . I wasn't interested in what was going on even though it was all to do with me

184 INT: yeah

185 CL: I was more interested in my son (2)

186 INT: did erm (2) what usually happens in these affairs is that each person has a little s- talk . so the social worker talks and the health visitor talks

187 CL: yeah I know (laughter) (3) yes and they all had a jolly good go at me . all they were talking about was my alcohol problem

188 INT: mm

189 CL: which seemed to be the main concern (2) and my non-ability to erm and they kept saying to me do you want to say anything (.) and I thought (.) well there isn't (.) really isn't nothing to say is there I thought (unclear)

190 INT: mm

191 CL: in fact in front of (.) if you're a certain type of person you can (.) talk to people in front of a crowd . but if you're not a certain type of person (.) you can't sit in front of the crowd and say exactly how you <u>feel</u> (.) you can't sort of say . no I think this is wrong . no I think that is wrong

In all that we have heard from Hilary she has concentrated on two situations: one, before intervention, where she was isolated without support and struggling to cope; two, where she is in a case conference with 20 professionals scrutinising facets of her behaviour and personality. Chapter 4 describes a case conference as experienced by a client who knew the system well. Hilary, however, presents a picture of alienation from the process. Rather than a process of support or assessment, she describes it as a trial in which guilt is inevitable: 'like a judge and jury on you', in which everyone is judging her and 'they all had a jolly good go at me' (cf. 'in the dock', Urek (2004: 7)). Faced with the strength and extent of this criticism, she reports feeling detached from the occasion, all her attention going to the co-present child (whom she hadn't seen yet that morning): 'they kept saying to me do you want to say anything (.) and I thought (.) well there isn't (.) really isn't nothing to say is there I thought' (turn 189) and 'I just wanted to pick him up and play with him . I wasn't interested in what was going on even though it was all to do with me' (turn 183).

Also the client's final turn underlines her sense of being situationally incapacitated when it comes to defending herself. What possible defence is there for a client in this situation? For those that do defend themselves and successfully articulate the caring-but-not-coping formulation, a rebuttal may be client-centred. However, it may be heard as inadequate by the institutional representatives because it is not child-centred (see Hall and Slembrouck 2001). The problem seems to be that, while child welfare intervention is propagated on the needs of the child, the parent experiences the attribution of responsibility as inevitably pointed at him/herself.

This is illustrated in another case we would like to draw upon briefly. Ray, Cheryl and two daughters are involved in an assessment process. They had reported to their health visitor concerns that their daughter Helen had been abused by someone outside the family and was displaying inappropriate behaviour. The health visitor suggested a referral to a counselling service, but the family found that this could only be accessed through a social services assessment. The parents had had previous experiences with social services and were worried about such an intervention. Like Hilary, the intervention was client-initiated, but the assessment comes to be focused on the parents' capacities (rather than the child's needs). These parents take this shift up as a criticism.

Interview 2 – extract 1

49 CL: it seemed to be questions almost leaning away from not helping Helen but helping me and her mum whereas we were saying well we've been on sort of parent refresher courses before and I was trying to say that's not the thing we want to look at (.) again instead of whereas we feel that Helen needs help it should be up to Helen at the end of the day to decide how she would like us to go about it

Perhaps because of their previous experience with social services, the father draws on a vocabulary of children's needs and children's choice in discussing the nature of the intervention. In this way, he is able to challenge the focus on the parents. This further highlights the dimension of institutional literacy. These parents also challenge the way in which the assessment process was being carried out.

Interview 2 – extract 2

54 CL: [. . .] halfway through when we had nearly finished the core assessment they quite rushed us to sign and they said ooh we'll make a quick photocopy (.) and then we were told it's going to be sent out to places like the schools and it had personal information about me and Cheryl that we didn't want us next door neighbours to know

55 INT: and they'd not made that clear at the beginning (.)

56 CL: they'd not made that clear at all at the beginning and as I said earlier you know this core assessment (.) I just forgotten my main point now (.) it was going to deal more with me and Cheryl and not with Helen and that was the first point that we brought up and they said no Helen would be our main sort of focusing point (4)

57 INT: and you didn't think that was made clearer at the time

58 CL: no

59 INT: when they were talking to you and you were explaining the problems did you think they understood what you were saying did they listen to what you said

60 CL: erm (3) they listened yes they listened erm

61 INT: right

(shared laughter)

62 CL: and it took a few sessions to get them to understand the point that had to be driven home (.) virtually with a stick before sort of well let's look at it further (.)

63 INT: what do you think it was they didn't quite understand

64 CL: (5) ooh (4) again our main one was how me and my partner would feel about this core assessment going out to other third-party groups other than you know social services or any other services who might need to know but (.) and it could be open to anyone you know schools should not have access to the full core assessment but certain bits of it which are relevant to them

The parents were able to challenge some of the processes. They resisted being rushed to sign the assessment document and they questioned whether confidential information should be sent to schools (turn 54). And yet, despite their familiarity with social services, they still report not knowing in advance how the process works (turns 54 and 58). However, unlike Hilary, they managed to put across their points of view, even though this was not straightforward: 'it had to be driven home virtually with a stick' (turn 62).

Interview 2 – extract 3

69 INT: when you were in the middle of this were there any particular worries about what may or may not happen you mentioned the fact that information might get to other people

70 CL: yes

71 INT were there worries about the way the process was being handled

72 CL: erm (.) my main concern is and it's cropped up before especially with social services is (.) you know we're reading these programmes and leaflets and get as much information before we make a step forward and obviously you know we've had a few bad experiences with social services but (.) with the problem with what Helen had or has (.) you know we decided that social services you know would be the right route to go down this time (.) and once they're involved sort of halfway through (.) as soon as you know I or both me and Cheryl feel it might not be the right . course we don't feel we could say no (.) we don't want to pursue this course we'd rather change avenue and maybe try something different (.) we feel that becomes less and less an option

73 INT: you can't say no

74 CL virtually on every visit you know to say stop it almost means we will intervene anyway and and that is a great deal of sort of pressure (.) and it's not a good footing it's not a good basis to try and form a team relationship within the family unit and get results which is what I want

Just as Hilary describes her powerlessness to stop the social services' intervention and the associated scrutiny by professionals, these parents describe the difficulty in changing the course of an intervention (turns 72 and 74). They, too, had asked for what they saw as a supported service, but were forced to undergo the consequences of that request. Understanding social work processes, they realised they had to cooperate with the assessment and imply that this was initially their choice ('we decided that social services you know would be the right route to go down this time', turn 72). However, what they experience next is the impossibility to keep control of the process: 'virtually on every visit you know to say stop it almost means we will intervene anyway' (turn 74). This is seen as not only inevitable, but reported as a poor basis for working together with the professionals.

Conclusion

This chapter by no means offers a widely sampled review of client perspectives in the area of child protection. However, detailed analysis of client talk brings out important points, which are corroborated by Urek's (2004) analysis. In particular, it reinforces a relational concept of the self, that is: that people's conception of themselves is a product of those with whom they interact on a regular basis (as opposed to a holistic concept of the self as locked into the individual; Gergen 1999). From the account it has been clear that Hilary can only gain a conception of herself as a good parent through those around her and the relational selves we have heard her report all seem to be largely negative – neighbours, her own parents, the boyfriend, the social workers, etc. In addition, what justifications does she bring in to say that she cares and that she is doing a good job?

There is the general claim that her son should be with his mother (as she said at an earlier point, 'crikey my child's going to another home when he should be with me' and 'he's kept away from me for so long . and I never did anything wrong' in extract 7) and there are quite a number of instances where a more positive self is presupposed but remains hidden because the mother is/was incapacitated during pivotal moments of assessment or decision-making. There are implications here from a policy and practice perspective. While Hilary is articulate and able to express a range of reactions to social services intervention, she feels excluded from decision-making and inhibited during pivotal moments of assessment. The Jones family, on the other hand, appear more institutionally literate and possess the necessary discursive resources to talk about interventions being 'child-focused' and rights to privacy. However, even they describe the inevitability of conforming to social services systems. Clearly, there are implications for concepts of 'parent participation' (see Artinian *et al.* 2003; Slembrouck 2005 on client literacy).

Parent participation approaches would presumably attempt to gain some agreement about the nature and the extent of child neglect as well as negotiate a finite-list programme of how someone like Hilary can become a successful mother. However, our analysis shows that the very process of locating problems within parenting capacities makes a mutually acceptable formulation difficult and results in attacks on the self and a sense of powerlessness to resist. Note in particular the prevalence of court metaphors in clients' accounts. Hilary's comments (not covered in detail in our analysis) that she doesn't know what she has to do to get her child back, that her visiting of various counsellors is somehow not enough: 'I've no idea what I've got to do to prove (.) I'm doing everything that they want me to do . but I don't know (.) anymore . what I can do any more to prove that I can have him back'. There is also an issue of power here: when can a client say 'I don't want this intervention any more', especially when they have initiated the contact with the social services.

Thirdly, the stigmatising effects on parents when children have been removed from their homes or when involved in other processes should not be underestimated. As Goffman (1990) points out, stigma always comes as an interactional plight. It is the plight of not being able to ignore a particular 'detail' or 'feature' in interaction; it is the pressure of having to explain oneself, and having to explain what 'under normal circumstances' is routinely taken for granted; it is the plight of being constantly talked about. Note how even this interview situation does not form an exception to this, as is testified in the client's turn in the final extract below. It comes at the end of the interview and the interviewer asks permission for an interview with the foster parents.

Interview 1 – Extract 10

354 INT: yes (4) erm do you mind if I go and talk to the foster parents (2)

355 CL: no I don't mind (3) you can have a good chat about me.

356 INT: I wouldn't I wouldn't particularly want to talk just about you I mean erm (.) what we want to talk to foster parents about is much more erm (.) how things have changed since they've been foster p- I have already spoken to but a different foster parent (.) and and we're interesting in

There is a need to understand and investigate the dynamics of stigma from a practice perspective. As we have argued in detail elsewhere (Slembrouck and Hall 2003: 60), the thrust of Goffman's analysis raises the question to what extent social work, rather than hearing parents' explanations as 'excuses to be ignored', can actively take on board and anticipate in interaction that parents will feel accused and will want to redeem themselves. Approaches which focus on 'finding solutions' and 'building on strengths' might point in this direction (Parton and O'Byrne 2000), as long as the professional strategy of undermining the client's parenting capacities can be held in check.

8 Justifying action in a public inquiry

In this chapter, we examine how categorisation and accountability are features of communication in an atypical encounter, the questioning of social workers as witnesses in a public inquiry. Whilst it is not an everyday occurrence for social workers, we suggest that such a setting highlights important features of the construction of social work formulations and justifications. In the public inquiry, the everyday routine aspects of social work become visible and open to the detailed scrutiny of critical observers, appointed committees and overhearing media audiences. Memos, dairies, case notes, etc. are examined and the professionals are required to justify their actions.

Public inquiries in the UK have been a frequent response to high profile tragedies and public concerns about social work and related professions, particularly in child protection. Parton (2004: 82) considers that '(public inquiries) have probably been the most influential factor in bringing about change'. Whilst such inquiries are usually concerned with a single case, the detailed scrutiny of the public inquiry reveals concerns which are seen to pervade professional practice in general and consequently engender wide-ranging criticisms. Lynch and Bogen (1996: 122) see the examination of witnesses in an inquiry as 'confessional disclosure' obtained through 'the rationality of interrogation'. The battleground for such exchanges in child abuse inquiries is the logic, evidence and reason of the professional.

We suggest that investigating the examination of the talk of social workers' witnesses in public inquiries offers opportunities for understanding the construction of social work talk, but such requires caution. First, it is typical of everyday practice that the talk, assessments, hunches and narratives of social workers move between various contexts – reports, meetings, casual conversations – as information is passed between various professionals and agencies. Such information flows are rarely made visible. The public inquiry lays bare such routine activities, because reports, file entries and actions are systematically examined and re-examined. This process is an example of 'recontextualisation' (Bauman and Briggs 1990; Baynham and Slembrouck 1999): events and characterisations are revisited and reviewed in new settings. At the same time witness and barrister are engaged in a process of post hoc co-construction (in ways similar to the policy interviews in Chapter 3): that is, re-visiting and re-defining the nature of the events and characters and turning them into new versions. Thirdly, what were previously instances in a flow of everyday routine activity are picked out and made into more concrete and (in)defensible entities. The atmosphere of scrutiny in the public inquiry also enables us to explore the efforts of witnesses to both produce defensible accounts and to adjust their own performance, a heightened sense of practical reflexivity.

However, as public inquiries involve a post hoc scrutiny of events and characters, we are a couple of steps removed from the direct study of everyday practices. Whilst the inquiry data offer opportunities for a detailed study of social work formulations and justifications, the pressures of the inquiry dialogues will heighten the degree of alarm. Given our orientation to the here and now of social work talk, the direction of our analysis will remain how justifications are constructed in the context of a public inquiry, without making links to 'what really happened' in the case selected.[1]

Managing categories of need and risk

The Victoria Climbié Inquiry (Laming 2003) took place in the UK between September 2001 and July 2002 and considered the circumstances of the death of a ten year old girl, Victoria Climbié. Victoria had arrived in London in April 1999 with her great aunt, Kouao. She was seen by a number of professionals over the next few months, admitted to two hospitals and was the subject of child protection investigations. However, no formal assessment was completed, no case conference had been organised and the case was given a low priority. She died in February 2000 and her aunt and her partner were convicted of her murder. It was only after Victoria died that it was established that Mrs Kouao was not her mother but a great aunt. The professionals had worked with the family on the assumption that she was the mother of the child (this is also apparent from the ways in which the professionals talk about the case). Following widespread media coverage of the trial, the government announced a public inquiry. There was considerable media coverage and the inquiry's proceedings were made available on the internet (http://www.victoria-climbie-inquiry.org.uk).

The analysis will concentrate on the construction and contestation of categories associated with social work in inquiry talk. The Children Act 1989 is the legislative basis for the provision of child welfare services in the UK. Implemented following child abuse inquiries in the 1980s, it sets out to balance the rights of families to be protected from unwarranted intervention and removal of their children, together with the state's responsibilities for protecting children. This results in two different responsibilities – to support families and provide services to help children's health and development, and to protect and rescue those children considered to be at risk of significant harm.

Whilst there might be considerable overlap between the notions of support and protection, policy-makers, managers and practitioners have tended to treat them as distinct. Estimates are made of those 'in need' and those 'at risk' (Her Majesty's Government 2003: 15), and procedures entail distinctions between how cases should be handled. Guidance such as that offered by the Child Protection Committee in Kent stipulates how social workers and their managers have to decide if a child is 'in need' and, if so, which services are required to address the child's needs (Kent Child Protection Committee 2005: para 3.12). The guide states:

> At the conclusion of the initial assessment, and in consultation with the Social Worker who undertook the assessment, the Duty Manager will make a decision about appropriate further action. This may be:
> – no further action is required
> – where core assessment judged not necessary – refer for specified service by an identified agency
> – child in need – multi-agency core assessment to be co-ordinated by Social Services
> – a section 47 enquiry to be initiated (see Section 8)
> – emergency action to protect child

Following an initial assessment, a child may be categorised as 'not in need of social services', 'requiring further assessment', 'in need' (section 17 of the Children Act) or 'at risk of significant harm' (requiring immediate 'emergency action' or 'requiring a section 47 enquiry' to decide if a child protection procedure should be initiated).

In everyday work, cases are categorised as 'section 17' or 'section 47' cases to denote the section of the Children Act 1989 or labelled as 'family support' or 'child protection' cases. In the inquiry data, it will be apparent that notions of what is a child 'in need' and a child 'at risk' form the basis for categorisations for social work interventions and the scrutinisation of accountable action by the barristers during public inquiry.

Examination of witnesses in court and public inquiries

There has been considerable research into the nature of discourse and inter-action in courts settings (for example: Cotterill 2003; Drew 1990, 1992; Ehrlich 2002; Gibbons 2003; Harris 2001; Locke and Edwards 2003). Public inquiries involve examination by barristers and have notions about what constitutes evidence (Atkinson and Drew 1979; Lynch and Bogen 1996). In the Opening Statement by the Chairman of the Victoria Climbié Inquiry (2001: 5), Lord Laming comments:

> I have decided that the Inquiry will be inquisitorial and not adversarial in nature. It is not like litigation, nor prosecution. It is an investigation.

Witnesses were required to make statements and were encouraged to seek legal assistance, however the role of such lawyers in the examination of evidence 'will be limited' (p. 6). In the inquiry, the witnesses were questioned by the inquiry barrister, followed by a short re-examination by the witness's barrister and sometimes additional questions by the chairman.

Corby *et al.* (2001: 137), however, notes 'an adversarial structure and style' to gathering evidence in the North Wales tribunal. Similarly Atkinson and Drew (1979: 106) note:

> Tribunals of Inquiry do not have defendants, at least not in a formal sense, though it is well known that questioning may often be intended not merely to find out 'what happened', but to blame a witness or show that he was at fault in some respect.

Whilst witnesses in public inquiries are not on trial, they can be subjected to questioning which goes beyond merely disclosing the facts, challenging their competency, plausibility and integrity. (Some of the social workers and police were dismissed or disciplined following the inquiry.)

The Victoria Climbié Inquiry is concerned with the failure of professionals to identify the signs of the child abuse, so the 'master narrative' (Lynch and Bogan 1996: 157) of the inquiry is what went wrong with professional practice. Furthermore, the regular occurrence of high profile child abuse inquiries since the 1970s has cast a general orientation to blame and accountability across public discourse on child protection (Parton 1991: 52). As Victoria was killed by her carers, barristers and witnesses take for granted that this was a child protection case and all earlier professional contacts with the case were subsequently seen as evidence that she had been abused all along – what Dingwall *et al.* (1983: 80) call 'a prospective-retrospective fashion'.

The organisation of exchanges in public inquiries has features which are different from everyday conversation. Atkinson and Drew (1979: 190) note:

> Examination is a massively predominant and prevalent form of speech exchange in most, if not all, types of court. So too is the pre-allocation of turns and types of turns (i.e., one, which are minimally recognisable as 'questions' and 'answers'), as are the kinds of actions done with such turns (e.g. accusations, denials, excuses, justifications, etc.)

Drew (1992) outlines the features of the examination of witnesses – turns are pre-allocated, the lawyer speaks first and controls topic selection; turns are organised through questions and answers, and the talk is designed to be overheard by a non-speaking audience, the jury or inquiry panel. Harris (2001) notes the fragmented nature of witnesses' stories, with little opportunity for extended narratives. Whilst turns may be designed as questions and answers, Lynch and Bogen (1996: 140–141) note that exchanges are organised as assertions or descriptions which witnesses are invited to confirm, challenge or otherwise respond to. Confirmation is preferred, and where there is a challenge, an account is required. Furthermore, questions are not seen in isolation but as part of an unfolding line of argument:

> Questions are designed and heard as part of a developing series, which is presumed to have a point or to be leading somewhere, namely, to a challenge

or accusation. Not only do interrogators and witnesses organise their actions in accordance with the above scheme; that they do is accountable and is an interactionally used feature of testimony.

The organisation of the questioning locates witnesses' testimonies within accountable formulations of appropriate and inappropriate practice, (in)correct decision-making, identifying failure and attributing blame, played out in terms of professional standards and departmental procedures.

A number of researchers have explored ways in which witnesses and barristers argue over categories and their attributes. In their analysis of the Scarman tribunal, Atkinson and Drew (1979: 126) observe how the characteristics and location of sectarian groups in Belfast are the subject of examination, what they call 'the religious ecology of the city'. Attributions are made about the intentions of the rioters and the adequacy of the police response is being assessed. Locke and Edwards (2003) investigate how President Clinton attributes particular mental states and psychological characteristics to Monica Lewinsky in his Grand Jury testimony. Lynch and Bogen (1996: 171) see the struggle between interrogator and witness as 'suggesting particular categorical identities' and actions within this frame have 'moral implications'.

We suggest then that the examination of witnesses in the Victoria Climbié Inquiry offers an opportunity to study the construction and negotiation of social work, with categorisation and accountability as central characteristics. We will investigate the examination of two witnesses, the social worker involved in the first social work contact with the family and the social worker with the longest involvement (we refer to them as 'the first social worker (SW1)' and 'the second social worker(SW2)').[2]

Examination of the first social worker

In the first examination we consider, the social worker was briefly involved with the family when they were homeless. What is at stake in the cross-examination is whether or not the social worker was treating this as a case of a 'child in need' and the necessary assessment which this required:

Examination 1 – extract 1
Day 5, Tuesday 2 October 2001
page 2
12   BAR: Thank you. You were however in 1999 in that
13   post?
14   SW1: Yes, I was.
15   BAR: And you had been in that post since June of
16   1998?
17   SW1: Yes.
18   BAR: Ms (name), looking back on your involvement in
19   the case of Victoria, are you now content with the
20   quality of the job you did?

21 SW1: In hindsight, no.
22 BAR: Can you tell us the respects in which, with the
23 benefit of hindsight, you are not happy with what you
24 did?
25 SW1: I thought that with the assessment framework,

page 3
01   if that was in place, we would have had time to have
02   interviewed Victoria more thoroughly.
03   BAR: So it is principally in the inadequacy of the
04   interview of Victoria that you think there was error?
05   SW1: Yes, and the resources that were available at
06   the time.

This is the opening exchange between the barrister (BAR) and social worker after establishing her employment record. Unlike the structure of setting up an accusation by first establishing the relevant facts and categories (Atkinson and Drew 1979: 115), the barrister begins the examination with an implicit accusation. The first question accuses the social worker of inadequate work: 'looking back on your involvement in the case of Victoria are you now content with the quality of the job you did?' Rather than an accusation of a specific mistake or incompetence, this question is cast in general terms asking the social worker to assess her work as a whole. It is unlikely that the social worker could respond in a positive way given the 'master narrative' of the inquiry (Lynch and Bogen 1996: 157): any potential mistakes are qualified as 'in hindsight', implying that at the time she probably saw her work as adequate and is now invoking a retrospective viewpoint. Drew (1990: 45) sees such repairs as 'close to the heart of the disputatious nature of cross examination and the struggle [. . .] about how to depict the events at issue in a trial'. When pressed she indicates that, had the 'assessment framework' been in place (a recent practice tool to guide assessments, Department of Health, Home Office and National Assembly of Wales 2001), she would have interviewed Victoria more fully. The failure was a matter of previous assessment processes rather than her failure to comply. She therefore mitigates attributions of poor quality work by locating her work in the context of work practices at the time. Locke and Edwards (2003: 245) identify normalising action in witnesses' testimonies.

The barrister however re-emphasises personal issues of 'adequacy' and 'error' (page 3, line 03–04). He uses what Cotterill (2003: 150) describes as a 'so summariser' glossing the gist of the previous statement. Cotterill sees this 'third turn strategy' as indicative of a power-asymmetry. In this way the barrister resists the social worker's attempt to avoid an accusation of error. The social worker agrees but adds that resources were also a feature, again locating causes outside her control. By beginning the examination in this way, both barrister and witness have invoked the master narrative of the inquiry: inadequate professional practice but viewed in retrospect.

After a couple of exchanges about the lack of resources to meet the pressures of work, the barrister establishes the social worker's initial contact with the family as a referral from the Homeless Persons Unit.

Examination 1 – extract 2

page 3

22   BAR: Your first involvement with Victoria and with

23   Kouao occurred on 26th April 1999, I think.

24   SW1: I received a phone call from (housing officer).

25   BAR: Is she at the Homeless Persons Unit of your

page 4

01   same Council?

02   SW1: Yes, that is true.

03   BAR: And as a result of that conversation, a form

04   was completed, and I wonder if I can ask you to have

05   a look at that form. I think it is known as the yellow

06   form in (district), and it is in volume 5, please, page 217.

07   The photocopy is white, but I think that is a yellow

08   form, is it not?

09   SW1: Yes, it is.

10   BAR: That is the Children's Services first level

11   assessment core form. It is completed, I think, on the

12   front page by (housing officer); is that right?

13   SW1: No, it is not.

14   BAR: Who completed that then?

15   SW1: I completed that.

16   BAR: Thank you. Certainly you completed the second

17   page, we can see that from the paragraph headed 'Details

18   of Reasons for Referral', where you write:

19   'Received a telephone call from (housing officer), HPU.

20   She informed me that the Homeless Persons Unit are

21   unable to assist Mrs Kouao and her daughter. (Housing officer)

22   would like SS' – Social Services?

23   SW1: Yes, that is correct.

24   BAR: – 'to undertake an assessment of Mrs Kouao's

25   daughter's needs.'

page 5

01   So from the very start you were being asked to

02   focus, were you, on Victoria's needs?

03   SW1: Yes, that is correct.

The barrister locates the initial work as a phone call and completing 'the yellow form', which is the first part of an assessment process, 'the Children's Services first level assessment core form'. The social worker's activities are portrayed as engaged in a bureaucratic frame of form filling. The barrister makes a series of assertions, with which the witness is invited to confirm or correct for an overhearing audience (Lynch and Bogen 1996: 140; Gibbons 2003: 153). Whilst such exchanges may

appear merely descriptive and uncontroversial, the selection of events and processes locates the social worker as engaged in the performance of purposeful action and, as such, she is depicted as an active subject in those events, limiting any excuse of merely passive involvement (Ehrlich 2002: 735).

The Homeless Persons Unit cannot help the family, presumably because they do not meet their criteria for being homeless, so the housing officer asks social services to assess the child's needs. The descriptions of the family unit are important here. For the Homeless Persons Unit the family is Mrs Kouao and Victoria, however the action by social services is justified in terms of assessing the child's needs. The shift in category from a homeless family 'Mrs Kouao and her daughter' to 'Mrs Kouao's daughter's needs' establishes both the nature of the social services' mandate as well as criteria for the assessment of their intervention. Being a child focused intervention, assessing Victoria's needs entails something different than dealing with a homeless family. The passage is in the form of reported speech (page 4, lines 19–25), quoting from the case file, and does not merely represent the view of the barrister.

At page 5 line 1–2, the shift from quoting the case notes to a direct question attempts to establish the social worker's mandate – a focus on Victoria's needs. Note again the use of a 'so summariser' to emphasise this orientation. There is also the use of an upgraded formulation 'from the very start' to locate the initial focus of the work and again the problem is personalised as the social worker's task 'you are being asked'. The sequence of questions/assertions ends with what might be heard as a challenge. The social worker's response, 'yes, that is correct', suggests she had not 'heard' it in this way.

The barrister extends the challenge at the end of extract 2 by outlining an alternative position, that Victoria was not a child in need.

Examination 1 – extract 3
page 5

```
04  BAR: When she gave her evidence yesterday, (housing officer)
05      said that that was not precisely her intention; she did
06      not see this as a child in need case at that stage, but
07      that is how you understood it?
08  SW1: Yes, for both Mrs Kouao and Victoria at the
09      time, to look at their housing needs.
10  BAR: Did you take the view from that early contact
11      that Victoria was at least potentially a child in need?
12  SW1: The information that I got from (housing officer) was that
13      Mrs Kouao had enough finance until 1st May, so I made an
14      appointment, I believe, on 29th April for her to come to
15      the office, for an assessment to be undertaken.
16  BAR: Do we see the fact that she has enough money
17      until 1st May recorded in the form?
18  SW1: No.
19  BAR: Is that recorded anywhere in the notes?
```

20   SWI: I do not believe so.
21   BAR: So that is something you remember now, is it?
22   SWI: About the money?

In her testimony, the housing officer had said that she did not see this as 'child in need case' to which the social worker agrees, shifting back to a formulation of a homeless family, 'their housing needs'. The barrister challenges this, suggesting Victoria was 'potentially a child in need', and that the social worker's initial contact should have been considering such a categorisation as a possible outcome.

The social worker does not answer this question and shifts to a different stance by indicating that the family had enough money for a few days. If 'Mrs Kouao had enough finance until 1st May' then they were not yet homeless and an appointment could wait. The financial circumstances of the family are an attribute of the category 'homeless family' rather than a 'child in need'. The barrister challenges whether this evidence of the family's financial circumstances appeared in the file, implying that it was produced at the inquiry merely as a defence against an accusation about the delay in the appointment date. Drew (1992: 480) notes how witnesses use a lack of recall to avoid confirming certain pieces of evidence. Here the barrister uses the problem of recall to undermine claims about matters not recorded in case files.

At this point the barrister has been unable to establish for the inquiry that Victoria was being considered a 'child in need'.

Examination I – extract 4

page 7

08   BAR: Did you see Victoria as potentially a child in
09   need within the meaning of that expression in the
10   Children Act?
11   SWI: What the department done, usually when people
12   presented and said that they did not have accommodation,
13   every child was taken as a child in need under
14   Section 17, as a whole.
15   BAR: So the child was viewed as a potentially
16   a child in need within Section 17?
17   SWI: Yes.
18   BAR: And that is presumably why you entered what you
19   did on page 220 in that bundle, in the 'Service and
20   Action Plan', where you have written, I think, 'Mother,
21   child (pending) homeless (see referral) child in need',
22   yes?
23   SWI: Yes.
24   BAR: And by both of those two entries you have put:
25   'Assessment to be undertaken by the DSW', presumably the

page 8

01   duty social worker?
02   SWI: Duty social worker.

03   BAR: So from that early stage, you saw the need for
04   an assessment of a potential child in need?
05   SW1: Yes, that is what usually was undertaken.
06   BAR: If a child is assessed to be a child in need,
07   would your Council invariably ensure that he or she had
08   accommodation?
09   SW1: Yes.
10   BAR: You arranged an appointment, I think, for
11   29th April?

After several exchanges about the recording of information about financial circumstances was recorded, the barrister repeats the question about Victoria being a 'child in need'. The question is slightly different. In extract 3, the question relates to 'early contact' and how the case was being handled, whereas here it is related to the social worker's viewpoint, 'did you see . . .'. It is also explicitly located within the Children Act, defining the legal mandate more precisely. In response, the social worker shifts the focus away from her work with Victoria to an institutional response, 'what the department done', and habitual stance, 'usually when people represent'. The legal mandate is accepted but qualified as 'as a whole', implying that this was an overall justification, not specific to this case. It suggests a rather different view of practice, in which all work in this type of case is justified under section 17 of the Children Act. This is in contrast to the barrister's suggestion that implementing section 17 requires specific actions, notably an assessment to determine if Victoria is a 'child in need'. The barrister ignores any such distinction and again deploys the 'so summariser' to establish that Victoria was being viewed as 'potentially a child in need'. The social worker now agrees.

The barrister again locates the social worker's action in the case records. He resists the social worker's institutional/habitual stance by personalising the action 'you entered' and 'you have written'. The references to both 'homeless' and 'child in need' confirm that the social worker's entries are orientated to determining if Victoria is a child in need. At line 3–4 (page 8) he sums up the social worker's view of what should count as 'an assessment of a potential child in need'. Whilst the social worker agrees, she reverts back to the habitual response, 'what usually was undertaken'.

The barrister now challenges any categorisation of a 'homeless case', by subsuming concerns about accommodation within the category of a 'child in need'. This time he uses the institutional voice. If the Council assesses a child as 'in need' then they would ensure that she has adequate accommodation. In terms of categorisation, homelessness is a potential attribute of the category 'child in need' and not a valid category in its own right. This juxtaposition between the case being one of a homeless family or a 'child in need' is revisited in later questioning.

The social worker became involved with the case again in June and an assessment had still not been completed. The barrister questions whether such delays are normal, to which the social worker responds by once again categorising the case as 'housing needs'.

Examination 1 – extract 5

page 21

22   BAR: Were you surprised that that had not already
23   been done, given that the need for it had been
24   identified at the end of April?
25   SW1: What, a full assessment?

page 22

01   BAR: Yes. You had made an appointment for an
02   assessment for 29th April, and here we were at the
03   beginning of June, and you were still being asked to do
04   an assessment. Did that surprise you, or is that normal
05   at (district)?
06   SW1: I think at the time it was quite difficult. We
07   usually assessed people via housing needs, rather than
08   being child focused.
09   BAR: You assessed people generally on housing needs
10   rather than being child focused?
11   SW1: Yes, at the time. It was quite difficult with
12   the unaccompanied minors and all the other people that
13   were coming in. Their need was – looked towards
14   housing needs.
15   BAR: Can you go back to page 166 in volume 5,
16   please?

The barrister's use of an institutional voice, 'is that normal in (district)', enables the social worker to avoid personal criticism. However, the barrister's repetition in lines 09–10 indicate some consternation and invites a further elaboration. Interestingly, the social worker uses the term 'child focused' rather than 'child in need', implying a flawed orientation to assessment in general rather than a selection between potential categories (you can be child focused in dealing with housing needs).

The social worker justifies such a situation on the basis of difficulties with these sorts of cases. Victoria's case is now categorised like other cases of homeless people and 'unaccompanied minors' who present themselves to social services, and the response is a concern with housing needs. Note how the social worker hesitates with the categorisation 'their need was [. . .] looked towards housing needs', suggesting some uncertainty as to whether this is a valid category (Drew 1990: 43) notes how witnesses tend to avoid such self-repair).

Towards the end of the examination of this witness, the barrister has still failed to establish whether this was a 'child in need' case.

Examination 1 – extract 6

page 50

05   BAR: Did you feel at that stage that you had carried
06   out an adequate assessment of Victoria's needs?

07   SW1: In hindsight, no, but when they presented,
08   I believed – duty social workers believed that they had
09   quite a good relationship at the time.
10   BAR: You mean Kouao and Victoria had a good
11   relationship?
12   SW1: Yes, at the time.
13   BAR: Was Victoria with her that day? Your notes are
14   at 154, if that is what you are looking for.
15   SW1: Thank you. I cannot remember.

The barrister again accuses the social worker of inadequate work. Again the agreement is qualified 'in hindsight' but the social worker now provides a different justification. The general view of the duty social workers was that there was a good relationship between Kouao and Victoria, further downplaying the view that Victoria was a 'child in need'. Note how this justification is hedged in terms of the context of this viewpoint 'when they presented'. Also the perspective is changed from a personal to a collective one, 'I believed – duty social workers believed'.

Examination 1 – extract 7

page 55

02   BAR: At the time that the case was closed, had you
03   ever spoken to Victoria?
04   SW1: Yes, I had spoken to Victoria.
05   BAR: When was that?
06   SW1: Usually during reception, or when they came in
07   to see other social workers.
08   BAR: When last, prior to closing the case, had you
09   spoken to Victoria?
10   SW1: I would not be able to recall.
11   BAR: The case was closed without a home visit ever
12   being carried out to Victoria, was it not?
13   SW1: Yes.
14   BAR: The case was closed without the assessment ever
15   being completed, was it not?
16   SW1: Although it was brought to the management's
17   attention about that, that it was difficult.
18   BAR: Would it be fair to say, Ms. (name), that this
19   case was closed without Victoria's future having been
20   determined or her welfare protected by (district)?
21   SW1: In hindsight, yes you can say that, but at the
22   time, she presented as a loving mother.
23   BAR: She had been referred to you by the Homeless
24   Persons Unit as a child in need; did you ever satisfy
25   yourself that she was not?

page 56

01   SW1: No, I would have needed complete information.

In summarising the social worker's involvement, the barrister sets up an accusation on the basis that the case was closed without the social worker speaking to Victoria, without a home visit and without an assessment having been completed. Such a list amounts to strong criticism. It challenges the tenets of good professional practice – talking to the child, a home visit, departmental procedures. Each item is prefaced with 'the case was closed . . .' establishing the list structure (Jefferson 1990). The social worker disputes the first of these charges but accepts the second and third. The resulting accusation at line 18 recruits agreement from the witness, 'would it be fair to say' and uses an institutional voice, 'this case was closed . . .' and 'protect by (district name)' rather than a personal criticism. Even so, the defence at line 21, contains a range of qualifiers, 'in hindsight' and veiled agreement 'you can say that', followed by a repeat of the depiction of the case as not a 'child in need', 'she presented as a loving mother'. The barrister ignores the earlier uncertainty about the appropriate categorisation for the final accusation; he is now stating firmly that Victoria had been referred as a 'child in need'.

   This examination of this witness started with a general accusation of poor social work practice but subsequent exchanges resulted in a dispute over the precise categorisation. The barrister advances a formulation of events in which the social worker was engaged in certain assessment processes to determine if Victoria was a 'child in need' as mandated by section 17 of the Children Act. Such practice necessarily involved certain features – completing an assessment, visiting the home, speaking to the child – which would decide if Victoria was a child in need. The implication is that, had a proper assessment been carried out, there would have been an opportunity to identify (and possibly prevent) the abuse that Victoria faced. The social worker resists this formulation. The case was essentially a homeless family with no evidence of other concerns – they had some money, there appeared to be a good relationship, Mrs Kouao presented herself as a loving mother. At the time there was no formal assessment system in place. Although the case involved a general orientation to Victoria being a 'child in need', this was like many other cases where the main priority was to sort out their housing needs.

   The barrister displays a formal notion of 'child in need' processes, the aim of which is to establish a clear categorisation: was Victoria a 'child in need' in which case appropriate services should have been provided? For the social worker, who is facing the everyday pressures of work, there is only a general orientation through the mandate of the Children Act.

   In summary, the examination of this witness was established with an ascription of poor practice, the master narrative of the inquiry. Notions of accountability are constructed by the barrister and defended by the social worker deploying devices of institutional voice versus personal agency, formal and everyday notions of professional practice, and retrospective viewpoints. Such exchanges involve the construction and contestation of categories of social work, in this particular case 'homeless families' as opposed to a 'child in need'.

Examination of the second social worker

The second social worker was responsible for Victoria's case for the longest period and was involved in what were seen as the key decisions, so the examination during the public inquiry took longer and was more complex than above. Here the category in dispute is why the social worker did not see Victoria as a child at risk of significant harm (requiring a section 47 inquiry). Briefly, the social worker was allocated the case after Victoria was admitted to hospital with scalding injuries. A section 47 child protection investigation was started but not completed after the social worker and police officer decided that there was no evidence that Victoria's injuries were caused deliberately. Perhaps more than in the first examination, the 'master narrative' is invoked: Victoria was being abused, the scalding was clear evidence of this and there were old marks that had been noted by the doctors. Here was an occasion where professionals should have recognised the signs and intervened. The examination concentrates on the decision to abandon the section 47 investigation and the elements of what constitutes a 'child at risk' are contested.

Examination 2 – extract 1
Thursday 22 November 2001
page 87
19   BAR: There is nothing to suggest any sort of
20   evaluation process of where you had got to.
21   SW2: There was no evaluation process.
22   BAR: Should there have been?
23   SW2: Definitely, yes.
24   BAR: That is an error by you, is it not?
25   SW2: I consulted with my managers at every

page 88
01   step of the way with Victoria's case.
02   BAR: That is slightly different, is it not? You
03   said to us earlier that reflection is important in
04   social work and you also said that there was not much
05   time for reflection in this office but nonetheless you
06   ought, ought you not, to have found time in a case like
07   Victoria's to make an overall assessment during the
08   course of your handling of it?
09   SW2: You are saying a case like Victoria's.
10   BAR: A case where initially there were child
11   protection concerns.
12   SW2: I believe I made that evaluation at the
13   start, when I received her file.
14   BAR: But not again thereafter?
15   SW2: Not again thereafter.
16   BAR: And should you have done?
17   SW2: I believe I should have done, yes.

In the first exchanges about the appropriate categorisation of Victoria's case, it is the social worker who challenges the barrister. As in the first examination, the barrister's initial challenge of the social worker's practice is criticism of her overall approach to the case, that there was 'no evaluation process'. He emphasises the importance of assessment 'in a case like Victoria's'. This might have been a passing comment but the social worker questions what he means by this. Now the barrister makes a clear categorisation, 'a case where initially there were child protection concerns'. Note how the barrister proposes a categorisation of the case which is less controversial; 'initially child protection concerns', and that there were 'concerns', not evidence. The social worker does not dispute this and accepts the criticism of inadequate evaluation.

Examination 2 – extract 2

page 101

```
06  BAR: From the time you received these papers
07  Ms. (name) you were taking part, were you not, in
08  a Section 47 investigation?
09  SW2: Yes, that is correct, yes.
10  BAR: Because child protection concerns were
11  immediate concerns from day one?
12  SW2: That is correct, yes.
13  BAR: So it is for you, is it not, from that moment
14  to make inquiry so as to ensure that Victoria is safe?
15  SW2: Those inquiries should be made as soon
16  as the referral is received on the Duty Team.
```

In this extract, the barrister uses a strong criticism which further develops the category of a child protection case. Note the use of the formal address to the social worker (line 7) and the reminder of the legal status of work in which she was now engaged – a section 47 investigation. Next some of the elements of such an investigation are spelt out, using a strong rhetorical figure (lines 10–11), 'child protection concerns were immediate concerns from day one', which is subsequently upgraded in the social worker's responsibility to 'ensure' Victoria's safety.

In terms of categorisation work, there is still no discussion of the characteristics which constitute a case which is 'clearly child protection'. Instead, the categorisation is formulated in terms of certain processes, implying that any case where there is a section 47 investigation is necessarily a child protection case – what Sacks (1992: 301) calls a category-bound activity. This can be contrasted with categorisation work where the properties of the categories are negotiated rather than the status of the category itself. At this early stage, both barrister and witness are sensitive to the categorisation of the case. Note how the social worker deflects responsibility for immediate action to the 'duty team', in the same way that the social worker in the first examination had invoked habitual processes.

The social worker is now questioned about how, having read through the file, she began to carry out the tasks set down at the strategy meeting. On August 3 the social worker was contacted by the hospital and informed that Victoria was 'ready for discharge'. The barrister spends some time examining what the hospital meant by 'medically fit for discharge', and how this affected the investigation. The social worker telephoned the nurse on Victoria's ward and asked to be sent the reports they had available. The barrister now summarises the material which she had at this point:

Examination 2 – extract 3

page 128

10 BAR: Let us look, in any event, at what material had
11 reached you by 3rd August insofar as it related to
12 physical abuse. You had the original referral sheet
13 from (duty social worker).
14 SW2: That is correct, yes.
15 BAR: You had the strategy minute meetings.
16 SW2: Yes.
17 BAR: You had the CP form, obtained that day, you
18 remind me.
19 SW2: Yes.
20 BAR: You had the body maps.
21 SW2: Yes.
22 BAR: You had (paediatrician's) concerns noted at least, as
23 we see them on page 65; yes?
24 SW2: Yes.
25 BAR: Six lines or so from the bottom:

page 129

01 'When she was examined Paediatrician (name) noticed
02 old injuries which appeared to be non-accidental.'
03 SW2: Yes.
04 BAR: And you had, you tell us in paragraph 85 of
05 your statement, Nurse (name)'s observations about old
06 injuries being NAI.[3]
07 SW2: Yes.
08 BAR: So there is a build-up of material there, all
09 of which suggests that the (hospital) had
10 concerns about non-accidental injuries.
11 SW2: Not specifically, no. I knew that (the
12 hospital) were concerned with old markings
13 which had been found on Victoria's body but nobody made
14 specific reference to these marks being as a result of
15 non-accidental injury.

The barrister asks the social worker to consider the evidence available to her on 3 August and how it suggests a categorisation of physical abuse, a much more specific category than 'child protection concerns'. The various documents are listed without acknowledging their content – the referral sheet, strategy meeting minutes, the child protection form and the body maps. The next item is the '(paediatrician)'s concerns'. They are quoted from the strategy meeting minutes (page 129, line 01–02) and describe the paediatrician noticing 'old injuries which appeared to be non-accidental'. This reported speech is presented as an observation from the doctor's examination and can be heard as indicating evidence of abuse. Quoted in this way it stands out from the rest of the material as the central event which led to the referral. However, given the nature of the investigation stage, the evidence is hedged: the doctor 'noticed' injuries which 'appeared to be'. It is not evidence of abuse but evidence of concerns that there might have been evidence of abuse. However, the use of 'at least' (page 128, line 22) implies that any reasonable person would see that there were concerns. The social worker's own statement mentions the nurse's observations, highlighting her orientation to signs of abuse.

The barrister is then able to summarise the situation, again prefaced by 'so'. Whilst maintaining the tentative nature of the evidence, his summary (page 129, line 08–10) aims to establish the current level of concern. It is a cumulative 'build-up of material', it points in the same direction, 'all of which suggests', and establishes the hospital as having a unitary viewpoint, 'the (hospital) had concerns'. It is not merely one doctor but the whole institution of the hospital. In response, the social worker contests the suggestion that the concerns pointed at a build-up of evidence and implies a category of non-accidental injury. She makes the contrast between 'old markings' and their cause being non-accidental injury. Although the hospital had observed the markings, they had not specifically suggested that they were caused by non-accidental injury. The social worker has reversed the barrister's implication: there were markings on Victoria that caused concern to the hospital but as yet no one had made the move to explain the cause of these markings as non-accidental injury. It is possible that markings had other explanations. The phrase 'nobody made specific reference to' (page 129, lines 13–14) is however a statement of omission and does not imply a reference to any particular hospital professional. The social worker had heard these observations but not received their explanation. This position of the social worker as a receiver and hearer of other people's observations and assessments is reaffirmed in the next exchanges:

Examination 2 – extract 4

page 129

16 BAR: Look at page 41 in volume 6. This is the
17 original referral sheet I think from (duty social worker).
18 SW2: Yes.
19 BAR: Halfway down that piece of text:
20 'The next day on Rainbow Ward the nurse bathed Anna[4]
21 and saw old marks on child's body. Up until then the
22 staff did not suspect physical abuse but since
23 witnessing the marks they feel sure they are
24 non-accidental. (Paediatrician) suggests that the marks look
25 like they were done by belt buckles.'

page 130

01   SW2: Yes.
02   BAR: So you had that much from the (hospital)?
03   SW2: In the initial referral, yes.
04   BAR: Paragraph 89 of your statement you say, first
05   sentence:
06   'Whilst possible emotional abuse was specifically
07   mentioned neither (nurse)'s notes nor the (hospital)
08   medical information referred to physical abuse.'
09   You see, what I am suggesting to you is you would
10   not expect Nurse (name)'s note to refer to physical abuse
11   because she was writing with respect to a request
12   relating to emotional abuse; do you agree with that?
13   SW2: I agree with that.
14   BAR: But the rest of the (hospital) material did on
15   a number of occasions refer to physical abuse including
16   the referral sheet which I have already taken you to, so
17   how can you write 'nor did the (hospital's) medical information
18   refer to physical abuse'?
19   SW2: The (hospital)'s medical
20   reports that were sent to me did not make specific
21   reference to physical abuse.

The barrister produced more evidence to support his contention that the evidence available pointed towards physical abuse by quoting from the referral sheet. In it, the nurse is described bathing Victoria and seeing 'old marks'. The pictorial display not only displays the life of the ward but presents their realisation process – at first they did not suspect child abuse but now 'feel sure' (page 129, line 23). The paediatrician is now able to suggest a cause: 'belt buckle' (page 129, line 25). After drawing the social worker's agreement (page 130, line 1), the barrister again uses an 'at least' formulation. The social worker retorts that this was at the initial referral, implying that such evidence was superseded by subsequent contact (page 130, line 3).

The barrister now quotes the social worker's statement back to her: although emotional abuse was mentioned, none of the hospital evidence referred to physical abuse. He suggests the nurse did not mention physical abuse, as she had been asked to report the emotional abuse (page 130, lines 10–12); however other material from the hospital referred to physical abuse on several occasions. The social worker's words are now put back to her to further undermine her position. Drew (1990: 49) notes the way that barristers are able to juxtapose prior testimony with present matters, displaying inconsistency often with damaging implications. It simplifies possible ways of viewing the case into two contrasting formulations, the preferred version of the barrister and the dispreferred version of the social worker.

The social worker's defence builds on seeing matters from a personal and hence restricted viewpoint. Whatever may have been said on other occasions, the information sent to her did not refer to physical abuse. It should be noted that earlier it had been reported that the social worker had asked the nurse to fax her all the information that they had. So the social worker appears to suggest that the information sent in this fax was the most up to date and represented the hospital's current view.

Examination 2 – extract 5

page 131
15 BAR: Did that taken in the round not lead you then
16 and there to start a full assessment of Victoria?
17 SW2: In order to begin a full assessment of
18 Victoria I needed a medical report which gave clear
19 diagnosis of non-accidental injury.

The barrister continues to demonstrate that the social worker's view of the case was at odds with the evidence from the hospital and changes the direction of the challenge. He again uses a summarising imperative, 'in the round' (page 131, line 15), requiring the social worker to take a dispassionate and eclectic view and to back it up with decisive action 'then and there' (page 131, line 16). Not merely has the hospital evidence raised concerns of physical abuse but those concerns were enough for the social worker to start a 'full assessment'. This is the stage in the child protection process where the social worker accepts that there is sufficient evidence to merit a wide investigation of the family's circumstances, gathering evidence from various sources, and clearly upgrading the status of the case.

The social worker responds with a minimal stance: to start a full assessment, she needs 'a medical report which gave clear diagnosis of non-accidental injury' (page 131, line 18–19). Such an orientation to evidence, assessment and action is at odds with the barrister's. He is promoting an approach in which the social worker gathers evidence and observations from others, and then makes the assessment of its significance so as to decide whether it constitutes enough of a case to warrant the application of a categorisation of 'serious concerns'. After this, appropriate action should follow. The social worker on the other hand requires that the medical staff provide evidence and observations, report them as concerns and establish a categorisation of child abuse. Only with a 'clear diagnosis' can the social worker act.

In summary, the construction and negotiation of Victoria as a 'child at risk' shows important differences to the early exchanges with the first social worker. There the exchange revolves around the two categories of 'child in need' and 'homeless family'; here at issue is when to apply a category of 'physical abuse'. The barrister constructs physical abuse in terms initially of processes, a section 47 investigation, a strategy meeting, and then the observations of doctors and nurses. The social worker resists the suggestion that this is enough for the category to apply and sees evidence in terms of how it is communicated. To establish a categorisation of physical abuse requires an implicit medical diagnosis, without which the investigation cannot proceed to the next stage.

Conclusion

In the case of this public inquiry, a dramatic outcome can be seen to temporarily 'suspend' routinely enacted definitions of what counts as an instance of a particular category. Decisions which were straightforward at the time are now unpacked and open to scrutiny. Categorisations established are being challenged. This chapter has explored categorisation and accountability in a public inquiry, in particular how a version of a child 'not in need', 'child in need' and 'child at risk' are constructed and contested. We have noted how the accountable nature of routine practice is undermined in a public inquiry by deploying the law and institutional guidance – assessing practice in terms of formal requirements. At the same time, the social workers can be seen to defend their actions through locating everyday routines and dilemmas.

In the second set of extracts, the barrister and social worker present two different versions of a child protection investigation: one more passive-reactive and one more pro-active. The matter does not receive a resolution during the stage of examination. The barrister questions the whole orientation that the social worker has adopted to the case, not merely mistakes but an inappropriate stance:

Examination 2 – extract 6

page 144

22   BAR: It sounds Ms (name) as if you
23   are simply the passive recipient of information that
24   you saw yourself as a collecting bowl into which people
25   could pour their observations about Victoria rather than

page 145

01   somebody going out on an investigation. Is that fair?
02   SW2: I knew that before I carried out the
03   investigation into Victoria I knew that I needed to have
04   all the relevant information.
05   BAR: Did you ask (the paediatrician): 'Is there any evidence
06   of physical abuse here'?
07   SW2: I did not ask her no.

The social worker concedes to the line of questioning but she does not, at this point, concede on record to its import. In addition to how the matter gets resolved in the interaction of the public inquiry, there is its subsequent uptake in the inquiry report.

Laming's recommendation in the chapter of the report which deals with hospital systems asserts that hospitals must introduce systems to ensure that no child about whom there are child protection concerns is discharged from hospital without a documented plan for the future care of the child. In the chapter on social services, the recommendation is bi-directional:

In any event it was (the first social worker)'s view that, if (the paediatrician) as a senior paediatric consultant who had examined Victoria had had any concerns regarding physical harm, she would have communicated those to her directly. I do not consider this an unreasonable view to take. On the other hand, it was (the second social worker's) job to pull together and evaluate all the information available and, if by some oversight, she had been given no explanation – or no plausible explanation – for all the marks on Victoria's body, she should have sought one directly.

(Laming 2003: 6.2.3.5)

The social worker does not take all of the blame: while it is accepted that the information supplied by the hospital would not have led the social worker to automatically accept that this was a child protection case, the report acknowledges the need for a pro-active response. However, unlike the barrister, such is not seen as the social worker failing to live up to role expectations.

In both pieces of examination, we have seen how social workers' views of what sort of case this is have determined both the nature of the assessment and the associated action. What has been at stake in the question/answer sequences has been how evidence points to one formulation of the case rather than another. Both witnesses have resisted the import of the barrister's formulations, so that, whilst in the end we know the case should have been categorised as child abuse, the justification for other categorisations has been maintained (arguably, this is also the case in the chair's report).

This highlights the difficulties of moving from bits and pieces of evidence to clear categorisations. Even marks on a child's body require plausible explanations and adequate framings to decide whether it was or was not physical abuse (e.g., a medical diagnosis in itself requires associated social explanations – cf. Dingwall *et al.* 1983: 52, and, we can add here: appropriate communicative stagings).

The implications for practice do not end here. At the beginning of the chapter, we quoted guidance from the Kent Child Protection Committee regarding how a decision should be made following an initial assessment. It is interesting to note that the decision as to what to do next is located in the duty manager and not the individual social worker. This suggests that social services have taken on board the issue but with a subsequent development that the responsibility for assessing information needs to be considered higher up the management scale. It would seem that it is no longer a matter of merely individual professional assessment.

9 Narrative transformation in media reporting

Whereas in the previous chapters we have concentrated on how social workers account for their practices, in this chapter we will be addressing accountability as a dimension of press coverage. More specifically, we will be examining the categorisation of a set of dramatic events in relation to accountability. We are interested in the way in which the death of a child well known to the social services is handled by different press outlets, both in terms of how the case is categorised and what forms of accountability are attributed to various parties.

It has widely been acknowledged by academics and journalists (for example Aldridge 1994, Toynbee 1999) that social workers often receive a particularly hostile press. Press coverage about social issues has a role in shaping public opinion to the extent that the ideas developed by the press are reflected in public attitudes. Social work is not experienced by a large proportion of the population, and it has been called an 'invisible trade' (Pithouse 1987) because it takes place in settings away from the public gaze. To many people, press reporting is perhaps the only source of information they have about social work. This media effect has been acknowledged by, for example, the Butler Sloss report on the Cleveland events, which devoted a whole section to the important role played by the media. As Franklin and Parton (2001: 234) note, 'the media do not simply mediate; they actively contribute to and influence politics, policy and practice'. The press reporting of social work is considered to have an important effect on the way in which social work is talked about at all levels, helping to shape the public mood, the political debate, social workers' morale and even the ways in which social workers relate to their clients (Franklin and Parton 2001: 235).

Before we move into the details of our case, we would like to discuss some of the research on the media coverage of child abuse. A particular reaction to such press reporting can be detected. Often this has been social work academics (e.g. Aldridge 1994) concerned to counter what they see as unfair criticism, as well as work by media researchers (e.g. Kitzinger 1996). Such work has sought to describe patterns of reporting but also to develop explanations for the nature of the coverage. Four themes can be identified.

First, there is the unrepresentative nature of the reporting. Although social workers work in a wide range of settings, a disproportionately large number of news reports concern social work with children. A study of almost 2,000 newspaper reports on social work in 1997 and 1998 (Franklin 1998) found that nearly three-quarters concerned social work with children. A preoccupation with child abuse made up almost one-third of the press reports, even though there have been a number of equally potential scandals in the care of elderly people (Aldridge 1999: 91). Child abuse reporting is itself predominantly concerned with the reporting of individual cases and disproportionately concerned with abuse outside the home, whilst the prevention of abuse or discussion of underlying causes receives little coverage (Kitzinger and Skidmore 1995).

At the same time, there has been work by researchers who resist what they see as not merely unrepresentative, but biased, reporting. Franklin and Parton (2001) report the highly critical character of much of the reporting, especially concerning child abuse where around 80 per cent was adverse coverage. Press coverage is depicted as 'vilification' (Aldridge 1994: 43), 'far from neutral and balanced', 'damaging' and 'misrepresenting social work' (Franklin and Parton 2001: 234 and 235). Explanations have been located in the explicit political agendas of newspapers, and in particular concerns about the role of the family (Aldridge 1999: 99–100).

This leads to a second theme: wider explanations of press reporting can be located in social work as 'a powerful symbol for state welfare' being at the same time ineffective and authoritarian. Franklin and Parton outline two polemical images of social workers: '(They are) denounced as wimps if they fail to intervene but decried as bullies if they intervene too much' (2001: 240). For them, because social work is seen to embody collectivist (rather than individual) and public (rather than private) solutions, it is at odds with the New Right agenda of 'rolling back the frontiers of the state' which emerged in the 1970s and 1980s, and this has been embraced by a number of newspapers.

A third theme has been to see the reporting of social work, and particularly child abuse, as a product of news values and the routine organisation of newsgathering. Newspapers are more interested in bad news. As Hills notes (1980: 19): 'child abuse makes for good copy'; it provides not only 'grisly details' but also the ritual humiliation of the social workers' failures. As Kitzinger (1996: 323) points out: 'Journalists are not in the business of faithfully recording the most common events, they are in the business of finding, constructing and selling 'news' in a particular way.' Kitzinger and Skidmore (1995: 52) observe that child abuse tends to be covered by generalist rather than specialist reporters, who are concerned with the news of the day rather than in-depth coverage. Furthermore, well-organised pressure groups or voluntary organisations are reported on favourably more often than public officials (Howarth 1991). Kitzinger (1996) analysed the media coverage of 'false memory syndrome' in the 1990s and concludes that it was influenced by what journalists saw as the credibility of particular groups and individuals, what she calls 'good sources and the power of personal accounts'.

Finally, the reporting itself has been identified as subject to constraints and fashions; in fact, Kitzinger (1996: 331) detects the development of 'child abuse fatigue' in the early 1990s. Two apparently contradictory practices are discussed. First, it has been noted that a particular orthodoxy to reporting child abuse has emerged, what is called an 'interpretative frame' (Aldridge 1999: 90) or 'media template' (Kitzinger 2000). Journalists tend to rely on returning to earlier reports to frame the present one, 'going through the cuttings' so that particular features and stereotypes are revised and re-established. However, at the same time, Aldridge (1994: 43) notes that some cases miss the media spotlight, with national reporting being either 'low-key' or even 'absent'. In the late 1980s at the height of child abuse reporting, cases with similar characteristics did not receive the same treatment as the Beckford, Henry or Carlile cases. Aldridge offers an analysis of the characteristics of cases which might have contributed to this, for example, if a defendant pleads guilty there is less material on the case available in court which the press can report. She also believes there has been a racist element.

A discourse approach to press reporting

Whilst press reporting about social work is not neutral, to add that it is 'biased' or 'misrepresentative' implies that there is a definitive version of social work and child abuse which the press choose to ignore. An alternative approach argues that many agents – legislators, campaigners, academics – as well as the press use the topic of child abuse to claim that they talk with authority about family life and the role of the state. It is worth noting that the political features which are revealed in textual analysis are important, not as specifications of the party political agendas of particular newspapers, but because specific (ideologically invested) versions of social reality are constructed and communicated.

To undermine one version of a topic whilst implying a better one has been referred to as 'ontological gerrymandering'[1] (Woolgar and Pawluch 1985). Their argument is that analysts study 'claims making' by ironising actors' assumptions about the objectivity of the entities they are studying, whilst leaving their own assumptions about the entities unexplored. Holstein and Miller (1993: 9) summarise the process:

> First, the analyst identifies particular conditions or behaviours. Then he or she identifies various claims made about these conditions or behaviours. Finally, the analyst highlights the variability of the conditions to which they relate. The implication is that since the condition is invariant, changes in the definition of the conditions must result from the social circumstances of the definers rather than the condition itself [. . .] this sort of analysis depends upon the 'objective' statement about the constancy of the condition under consideration in order to justify claims about the shifting definitional process.

This is seen as 'selective objectivism': some features are promoted as contingent and a result of vested interests, whilst other features are objective and unchanging. Woolgar and Pawluch (1985) consider that for social construction analysts there is no way out of this dilemma, and we do not propose to offer a solution. Troyer (1989: 44) suggests that we suspend:

> the issue of whether or not there is an external world and arguing that social problems researchers should look at how the agreement arises that there is a

social problem. . . . The definition itself is secondary: the primary concern is the methods (activities) used to create the problem.

So, in keeping with our approach to discourse analysis in this book, we will resist suggesting that one version of social work or child abuse is preferable to another. Instead, we will focus on how the media texts make available certain versions of social work and child abuse. We will not develop a view of the press as biased or unsympathetic since all reporting on social work is concerned with persuading audiences, constructing versions of families and professionals and allocating appropriate blame and responsibility.

A number of analysts have identified discursive devices and concepts, which can be used to analyse media reports. Wortham and Locher (1996) identify the concepts of 'voice' and 'ventriloquation' in the work of Bakhtin. This refers to the way in which writers are able to put words and ways of speaking into the mouths of the people they are reporting. By 'voice' they mean the way in which subjects are provided with particular attributes and social positions, and by 'ventriloquation', they mean the way the author uses phrases which are aligned with or distanced from the character. Central to the work of Bakhtin is the way in which such voicing is inevitably evaluative, the way in which it comments implicitly or explicitly on the social world and moral character of those subjects. Here we will concentrate on the way in which news reporters represent, juxtapose and evaluate different positions and perspectives of a child abuse case.

A particularly important way in which writers and speakers depict others is in the reporting of their speech. Reported speech has been the subject of considerable interest, with both direct and indirect speech report seen as opportunities for representation and evaluation. Following the work of Bakhtin and Voloshinov, in one sense all speech is seen as coming from another:

> All words have the taste of a profession, a genre, a tendency, a party, a particular work, a particular person, a generation, an age group, the day and hour. Each word tastes of the context and contexts in which it has lived its socially charged life: all words and forms are populated by intentions.
>
> (Bakhtin 1981: 294)

The words chosen to depict and describe people and events come with the 'taste' of their previous uses in other contexts. Even if the exact words of the other are reported, the way in which the words are contextualised, linked to other words, mimicked and paraphrased enable the writer/speaker to comment and evaluate. In relation to writing, Leudar and Antaki (1996: 11) see such process as 'co-authoring':

> This means that the reporter animates the reported talk. If one accepts the voice as an integral part of the talk, then the reporter co-authors the report.

In other work Leudar (1995) notes that so-called direct reports in the media involve the collage of what was said at different times in the original talk.

Another way in which a reporter can influence the voicing of the report is through contextualisation. The actual occasion of an utterance cannot be reproduced; so it must be reconstructed in the report (Tannen 1986, Slembrouck 1992). The reported words might be set within a context by providing information about the background of the case or the circumstances of the telling (cf. Hall *et al.* 1999a).

These concepts offer powerful devices for the analysis of media reporting of child abuse by concentrating on a detailed analysis of the reports themselves, rather than speculating about intentions behind them.

The Stephanie Fox case

In March 1990, Stephen Fox was found guilty of the murder of his three year old daughter, Stephanie. The family were well known to the welfare agencies as a result of previous injuries and Stephanie had been in the child protection register of the local authority for two years. After the trial, an internal inquiry was set up and reported in June 1990. Our analysis will be concerned with reporting at various points in the chronology of the case and across four sites – the national press, the local press and the professional press.

National press (broadsheet and tabloid)
19 Aug. 1989 'Death of child in care sparks inquiry call' (*Guardian* p. 11)
31 Mar. 1990 'Father gets life for killing girl' (*Independent* p. 2)
— 'Drunken father who scalped daughter gets life' (*Daily Telegraph* p. 3)
— 'Murdered girl was in danger all her life' (*Daily Mail* p. 9)
21 Jun. 1990 'Cash curbs played part in abused girl's death' (*Independent* p. 3)
— 'Social workers failed to save battered girl' (*Daily Telegraph* p. 3)
— 'Poll tax cut 'led to death of tot'' (*Sun* p. 17)
— 'Cash cuts linked to child's death' (*Daily Mirror* p. 2)

Local press: *Wandsworth Borough News*
11 Aug. 1989 'Father charged with murder of daughter' p. 1
18 Aug. 1989 'Father charged with daughter's murder' p. 1
30 Mar. 1990 'Father denies murdering daughter' p. 28
6 Apr. 1990 'Father gaoled for life for daughter's murder' p. 28
— 'Inquiry launched into child murder' p. 28
— 'Learn lessons from Stephanie's murder' p. 6, Comment column
22 Jun. 1990 'This must not happen again' p. 1, Lead story
— 'Glaring errors in care' p. 8, Comment column
29 Jun. 1990 'Fifty children at risk in Wandsworth'

Professional press: *Community Care*
10 Aug. 1989 'Inquiry follows death' p. 12
05 Apr. 1990 One para coverage in 'In Brief' column p. 7

28 Jun. 1990   'Action on child abuse', Comment column p. 11
—   'Staff increase needed to tackle rise in child abuse' p. 4
—   'Cuts contributed to child's death' p. 5

For purposes of analysis the data will be organised along the following events:

1   When the case first broke, August 1989: *Guardian, Wandsworth Borough News* and *Community Care.*
2   When Stephen Fox was convicted of murder, March 1990: national, professional and local press.
3   When the inquiry reported, June 1990: national, local and professional press.

We pose four questions: (1) Which events do the media cover? (2) What is the nature of the coverage at each stage: what elements of the story are selected and how is the selection categorised? (3) What transformations take place at the next stage: which elements are added and which are omitted? (4) How does this narrative transformation enable different agents to make claims about definitions of reality and the projection of certain causal links? A child abuse case goes through narrative transformations as different discourses are deployed in the story. We will be particularly interested in how different voices appear in the texts and how these claim (or are bestowed with) credibility and authority – journalists, neighbours, social workers, solicitors, team managers, directors of social services, doctors, police, judges, inquiry chairpersons, academics, etc. The metaphor of a 'transformer' which transforms an electric current to a different and higher voltage is useful here. The analysis will link into the overall themes of the book, namely, the categorisation of events and characters and the allocation of blame and responsibility. Four newspaper items have been included in the Appendix and will be analysed in greater detail.

Stage 1: Stephanie's death

Stephanie Fox was killed in August 1989. Her father Stephen was charged and remanded in custody following a court hearing. At this stage, coverage appears to be limited, without unanimity about the status of the case. The events are reported by one national paper, the local paper and the professional journal.

Local press

The local paper, the *Wandsworth Borough News* (*WBN*), reports Stephen Fox being charged and remanded at the first two court hearings on the front page. There are quotes by the police and the pathologist describing the cause of death as head injuries, but there is no comment on social services' involvement in the case.

Professional press

The *Community Care* (CC) item is headed 'Inquiry follows death'. It also reports the murder but notes that Stephanie was 'in care and living with her mother'. Aimed at a professional audience, it outlines the details of an inquiry, as reported by a spokesperson for the social services department. The reaction can be seen as proactive and rational – the inquiry will be 'urgent and thorough', oriented to 'establish the facts', etc. – possibly reassuring the professional reader that the department is acting to head off criticism before the case hits the headlines.

National press

The *Guardian* piece (see Appendix 2) is published nine days later and provides a range of voices, with an implicitly critical tone. This news item reports a hearing at the juvenile court, in which the mother is attempting to have the other children returned home. Given the different court arena, the names of both child and father are withheld 'for legal reasons', however, perhaps to make up for this absence, all the key professionals are quoted and named. Both the heading, 'Death of child in care sparks inquiry call', and the first quotes are from the magistrate who describes the case as 'horrifying' and calls for a 'penetrating inquiry'. Two contexts are described. The first details the murder through the words of the police, describing the conditions found in the flat and state of shock of Stephanie's sisters. The mother's voice appears in indirect speech, explaining how she had left the family to attend a family party. A second context provides a history of previous child abuse incidents – another child in the family had died, earlier injuries to the children and Stephanie being made the subject of a care order with the other children placed on the child protection register. This context is provided through an unidentified voice – 'The court was told [. . .]'.

At the end of the piece, the social worker is named and quoted. He had recorded other incidents of injury in the family but accepted the mother's explanation as accidental (as it was supported by a doctor). In the final sentence, the social worker is reported:

> Mr (name social worker) said he had not much experience of such cases but that he had said this to his superiors.

The social worker is not named nor quoted in any future report on this case, so it is interesting to study this particular report. It relates to a custody hearing in the juvenile court (now called the family court) following measures to remove the other children from the home. The mother has applied to have them returned home. There are restrictions on the reporting of such proceedings, notably anything which might enable the children to be identified (Children Act 1989, section 97–2). These restrictions will only be lifted in high profile cases. The use of the phrases like 'the court heard [. . .]' and direct and indirect reported speech locate the journalist in the court hearing, a third context. The journalist is the paper's

'Social Services Correspondent', so this report could be seen as a result of particular investigations and contacts.

We would suggest that this report makes available both a categorisation and blaming even though it is not explicitly 'hostile' to social work. The article's headline constructs a categorisation of death of a child in care using the voice of a magistrate. Reports which blame social work tend to draw on the trial of the murderer, but as yet no trial has taken place. The use of 'allegedly' is a common method of making a point appear true whilst acknowledging that it is not yet proven, yet one reason given for not granting custody is that the father 'may get bail'. Other familiar features of child deaths are present in the report – the detailed descriptions of the police, the reports of previous examples of death and injury in the family, all help to construct what Dingwall *et al.* (1983) call a retrospective-prospective, that is, a pattern of child abuse that was clearly present all along. Here we see an example of 'epistemic modalization' (Silverstein 1993) since the context of the pattern of child abuse, 'the narrated events' in the news item, is juxtaposed with the context of the murder. From the privileged position in the courtroom, the reporter is able to make the connection appear obvious.

The quotes from the social worker at the end of the news item constitute a blaming: it includes both an account and an excuse. Its placement after the depiction of the pattern of child abuse is heard as a possible reason for the failure to detect and categorise child abuse. His comment that his superiors were aware of his inexperience is heard as an 'excuse', spreading the blame to social services more generally and deflecting an assessment of an incompetent worker. As Potter and Wetherell (1987: 75) note, excuses are accounts which accept responsibility but claim mitigation from blame.

The piece ends with no commentary, yet we would suggest that the structure of the report has enabled the reader to make the connections – murder of child in care living at home, terrible conditions, previous knowledge of abuse, inexperienced social worker. And yet this is a case which has not yet come to court, the information used comes from the custody hearing. We would suggest that the nature of child abuse reporting in the late 1980s in the UK had become such a 'media template' that even a broadsheet newspaper could construct a typical child abuse tragedy from atypical sources.

In summary, there has been rather limited coverage of the Stephanie Fox murder at this stage, with only the local, professional and one national paper covering the case. Furthermore, there is no unanimity as to the status of the case – for the *WBN* it is a child murder, for *CC* it has the potential to become another embarrassment for the profession requiring a strong response and for the *Guardian* it is a rare opportunity to report a social worker incriminating himself.

Stage 2: Stephen Fox is tried and convicted

Stephen Fox was tried and convicted for the murder of Stephanie in March 1990. Inevitably, the reporting after conviction will focus on the detailed evidence which appeared at the trial, including gruesome aspects of the assault, but at the same time,

information. The implication is that the *Daily Mail* chose to highlight social services' culpability, by adding 'colour' to the 'hard news'; that the details of previous social services' action are not facts but a form of embellishment (in her view, style is defined as editorial policy and market niche, made possible through a 'causal model embedded in the narrative' (1994: 64)). Whilst there is much more detail in the *Daily Mail*'s account compared with other national newspapers at this stage, the other reports chose to report details of the murder in such a way as to categorise the case in a particular way – there is no definitive version of the 'facts'. Furthermore, we have already noted that the earlier *Guardian* report also made available a categorisation of child abuse and a potential blaming, with what must be a different editorial policy than the *Daily Mail*. We would suggest that it is the organisation of the report at various levels of textual formu-lation, which enables facts and events to make available categorisations, blaming and causal models (Bell 1991). Work on narrative by White (1980: 13) has noted that fragments of information can become a story when they are 'emplotted' – 'if by plot we mean a structure of relationships, by which the events contained in an account are endowed with a meaning by being identified as parts of an integrated whole'.

We would therefore question the distinction between hard news and colour, but suggest instead that accounts are organised in terms of categories and blaming/ responsibilities.

Local press on the conviction

The *WBN* provides detailed coverage of Fox's conviction on the back page and in the editorial comment (6 April 1990). Like the national press, it is concerned with both the horror of the killing and social services' culpability. Two reports on the back page separate the two forms of categorisation.

The top piece is headed 'Father gaoled for life for daughter's murder'. It describes the nature of the murder (much is repeated from the report of the trial on 30 March). In addition, there are conflicting depictions of Stephen Fox's character from his defence counsel and neighbours, the former that he is 'not a sadistic father' and the latter that he 'is a weasel of a man who likes to prove he's tough by hitting little children'. This item then is concerned to extend the depiction of the 'monster' and does not mention social services' involvement. Being a local paper, more of this report includes local features – for instance, street and hospital names and direct quotations from named neighbours. Below the item is a second item, headed 'Inquiry launched into child's murder' (see Appendix 2).

This item is quite different both in tone and orientation and is almost word-for-word the same as the editorial comment on page 8, headed 'Learn lessons from Stephanie's murder'. The difference between reporting a story and editorial comment is normally well-established with the former seen as 'reporting' events and the latter 'commenting' on their significance (Bell 1991), but this may apply less strictly in local newspaper reporting. In this paper, the report on social services' involvement on page 28 is clearly a comment piece. Indeed the only difference between the editorial on page 8 and the report on page 28 is that the three 'recommendations' at the end of the report are prefaced with 'We put forward a few suggestions'. Let us quote one of these: 'We can suggest that social workers must not take incidents in isolation, particularly where there is a history of unexplained injuries to the child'. This is language normally associated with comment pieces.

The editorial comment and report on the back page are set up in a similar way to the *Daily Mail* article. There is no mention of the murder. Stephanie's sad life is described, followed by considerable comment on the failure of the agencies. There are also important differences. First, there are no quotes from 'private reports'. Second, social services are mostly grouped with other professionals: police, doctors, health visitors and the NSPCC, depicting the shared responsibility of agencies. Third, the reader is led through local procedures of professional decision-making. Professionals 'visited regularly', 'they saw bruises', 'they held case conferences', 'they monitored the situation'. Fourth, the professionals' failure is clearly structured around mistaken thinking:

> But they continued to follow the fashionable dictat that a child is best off with his or her family. No matter what sort of life that child is given.

The list of 'talking' and inaction is then contrasted with a period which the child spent in a foster home (with no information of dates or length of stay). It appears in stark contrast with the horror of the abuse at home. The flow of events is stopped and the article draws on a pictorial imagery:

> Suddenly there were no more bruises or bite marks. No more 'accidental' scald marks. Suddenly Stephanie stopped banging her head against walls – a classic sign of mental disturbance.

However, temporal sequence returns: the child goes home 'and it all started again'. Such a contrast enables a strong critique of professional thinking which favours the family unit over the child's best interests. Unlike the *Daily Mail*, the blaming here is less on failure to act on the information available than it is on action guided by a flawed ideology. A perceptive reader of the newspaper may perhaps be surprised that in the first four reports on this case, there was no mention of social services' involvement, but when it does appear, it comes with strong overtones of comment.

Professional press on the conviction

In *Community Care*, a small item appeared in the 'In Brief' section without a heading, again starting with the launch of an 'independent inquiry'. The murder is described as a 'horrific drunken attack' by her father. However, a sense of this being part of a pattern of child abuse is suggested by noting the long-term involvement with social services ('in care but living at home'):

Stephanie aged three had been battered and beaten by her father, Stephen Fox, whilst she was in the care of Wandsworth SSD but living at home.

Furthermore, the report does not directly blame social services in as much as it highlights unacceptable professional practice: that a child in care but living at home died, that a pattern of child abuse remained undetected by social workers despite their formal responsibility for the child. The professional reader can hear a case which needs to be explained, with all the hallmarks of professional negligence highlighted in earlier child abuse inquiries. The news item prepares the social work audience for future criticism, but at the same time it looks forward to the upcoming public inquiry to address certain questions.

In summary, at this stage, then, the case has become one of a particularly violent child murder and one in which social services are involved. The monster of the drunk and violent father is the main characterisation in most of the coverage, but in some reports, the *Daily Mail* and *WBN*, the case has been transformed into one of serious social services failure. For the *Daily Mail* it is a failure of social services to recognise and act on the obvious signs of an ongoing pattern of child abuse. For the *WBN* it is a more general failure of social services impaired by a flawed ideology. The self-incriminating voice of the inexperienced social worker in the *Guardian* has not reappeared. The social worker's voice in the *Daily Mail* appears rather helpless, expressing concerns but somehow constrained from acting on them. The social work voice in the *WBN* is more bureaucratic, following procedures, being 'well-meaning' but hamstrung by 'diktats'. These are not so clearly the messages of professional incompetence and negligence suggested by other research, but social workers caught in debilitating systems and ideologies.

Stage 3: The inquiry report

When the public inquiry reported in June 1990, there was widespread coverage in the national, local and professional press, but with very differing orientations.

The national press

All the national press shift the emphasis of the blame away from both the murderer and the social workers towards the local authority policy of reducing services to maintain a low tax regime – noted by all the papers as 'the lowest in England at £148'. However the emphasis is different in each report.

The *Daily Telegraph* (21 June 1990) provides the most comprehensive report. It is headlined: 'Social workers failed to save battered girl' and begins the report with failure to act despite knowing the facts, in a manner similar to the earlier *Daily Mail* report. However, the second paragraph notes that the inquiry report said that 'a shortage of staff may have contributed'. Two main criticisms of practice are reported – that there was no master record of the child's injuries and at no time were the police asked to investigate. But most of the report is concerned with shortages of staff, lack of cover for illness and no day-nursery places, which are reported as 'a matter of policy when savings were required'. Such shortages are linked directly to the case with quotes from the chair of the inquiry that a day nursery was not found for six months and there were delays in transferring the case when the experienced social worker left. Blame is directed away from the professionals:

> '[. . .] generally the concern and commitment from all of the staff from each of the agencies involved has impressed us all.' Prof Stevenson said that nothing the inquiry team had seen would have led to the inescapable belief that the murder might have been predicted.

There are further quotes from another member of the inquiry team and the local union representative about the effects of cuts on services by both national and local government. These are contrasted with the director of social services' indirect speech accepting some blame, 'admitted' but saying that staff levels are better than in other parts of London.

The reader of the *Daily Telegraph* may be surprised by the contrast between the headline and the body of the report. The social workers are first blamed for failing to act when they had the facts, but for most of the report it is the council's policy of cuts which are blamed. There are a large number of direct quotes for Professor Stevenson and another member of the inquiry panel is quoted seeing staff shortages as a general trend with widespread implications. Yet, the report is more circumspect than other national newspapers in making a direct link between the cuts and Stephanie's death. It uses the phase 'may have contributed to her death', and the quote by the director about higher staff levels rather undermines the case of shortages. The paper therefore resists using its own voice to apportion blame, instead leaving the reader to judge between the veracity of the Inquiry and the director of social services.

All the other national papers explicitly head their report in terms of a link between cuts and Stephanie's death, with more direct attributions: 'Cash cuts linked [. . .]' (*Daily Mirror*), 'Cash curbs played a part [. . .]' (*Independent*), 'Poll tax cut "led to death of tot"' (*Sun*). However, different voices are used to establish the link. The *Daily Mirror* quotes extensively from the local professional union official. The *Independent* contrasts the voice of the union official with a statement from the director of social services about not cutting resources for child protection. Another difference from all the other reports is that at the end there is a quote by the opposition social services spokesman, which reinforces the headline:

> This tragic case shows that you pay too high a price for the lowest poll tax in England.

Here the link between Stephanie's death and the low poll tax is made most directly, especially when compared to the newspaper headlines, 'linked to' or 'played part'. Yet it is not a direct blaming, as would be the case for example in 'low poll tax [2] caused death'; rather, the focus is on the actions of the council. The consequences of a policy aimed at achieving the lowest poll tax are that such deaths are made more likely. This new voice in the *Independent* extends its sources beyond the quotations obtained from those directly involved, thus adding a wider dimension to the story of Stephanie's death. Finally, the report in the *Sun* makes a direct link between the cuts and Stephanie's death, using the term 'led to'. It also makes an interesting distinction between the professionals and the council:

> Social workers knew she was at risk and wanted her safely looked after at a day centre. But the London Borough of Wandsworth, where Stephanie lived, reduced its care facilities on the way to setting England's lowest poll tax.

We hear the social workers as separated from the council and their ambitions to protect Stephanie as frustrated by cuts.[3]

In summary, the coverage in the national press at this stage is through the voice of the inquiry report, turning the blame away from both the murderer and the social workers and towards the council's cuts policy. However, there are important differences between individual papers with different voices being privileged and different methods of apportioning blame being applied. The inquiry report is provided with full authority to assess the facts and apportion blame, and none of the papers make a bid to provide a more privileged reading or make wider claims. Shifting blame away from the social workers can be exemplified by the way in which the *Daily Telegraph* refers to the head of the inquiry as 'Prof. Olive Stevenson, a former social worker now at Nottingham University'. There is no suggestion that being a former social worker reduced her authority and her reported quotes are the most extensive.

Local press

Coverage in the *Wandsworth Borough News* was extensive and was continued for several weeks. On 22 June, the *WBN* presents the inquiry report on the front page with the headline 'This must not happen again' and in an editorial comment on page 8 headed 'Glaring errors in care'. Unlike the national press, the report is predominantly concerned with professional and bureaucratic failure, and less with cuts in services. One particularly strong criticism expressed in the editorial and which has not appeared in any of the other papers notes that visits to the family were not carried out because of industrial action. This is followed by a strong criticism:

> [. . .] social workers must look closely at their consciences that a child is not going to be at risk when they decide to take legitimate industrial action.

The social workers are not only flawed in ideology, and failing in their procedures, they are also accused of serious moral misjudgements.

The following week another item in *WBN* (29 June) considers the overall situation of children on the child protection register without an allocated social worker. The item is headlined 'Fifty children at risk in Wandsworth'. An earlier report which stressed that Stephanie Fox should have been taken into care is revisited in a longer dialogue with the chair of the social services committee. The chair and the director of social services accepted that some cases were unallocated. However, there was a recruitment campaign to attract more staff, there are no very young children without a social worker, figures in a neighbouring borough are worse. Following these quotations, an unnamed source is reported:

> A normally reliable source within the council said that families without an allocated social worker would 'get what care is available – but it will be ad hoc'.

At the end of the piece, the Councillor is quoted countering both the claims of the cuts in services and the criticisms of the paper's earlier editorials that Stephanie should have been taken into care:

> We spent forty-seven million pounds on social services last year in Wandsworth. There were no cash cuts and we spent thousands trying to help the Fox family. The only thing that could have saved that little girl is if we had removed her from her family – and after Cleveland that is no longer publicly acceptable

The ideology of maintaining children who are at risk in families which had been the centre of the *WBN*'s criticism is allowed to be brushed aside in an unquestioning way. The claim is that, following the Cleveland inquiry in which children were seen to have been unnecessarily taken away from home, such policies are no longer 'publicly acceptable' and blame is thus shifted, away from the professionals and cuts, to received public opinion.

Professional press

There is widespread coverage in *Community Care* of 28 June 1990 (see Appendix 2). Like the national press the article on page 5 picks up the cuts theme with its headline: 'Cuts contributed to child's death'. However, the coverage of the inquiry findings is highly detailed and concentrates more on aspects of professional practice than on the cuts. The cuts perspective is displayed in the headline and first paragraphs. The rest of the report highlights professional failings. The phases are also less directly deterministic than those used in the national press: 'cuts contributed' and 'must take some of the blame', implying the role of other causalities. The trade union's claims of more planned cuts are reported but these are contrasted with denials from the chair of social services committee.

The majority of the item covers professional failings, including some features not mentioned in the national press. For example, the period without a social worker was characterised by transferring the case between offices, and is noted as a bureaucratic and boundary problem typical of pressurised work allocation systems which are oriented towards shifting work on to others. There is even a direct criticism of the social worker's competence, his 'slowness in acting' and 'for failing to give sufficient weight to the views of the day nursery'. The final comment is that professionals are warned that they:

should recognise the significance of persistent parental denial of any responsibility for injuries to their children.

This last comment underlines the way in which the Community Care report is orientated towards professionals taking note of the criticisms of an inquiry led by a respected social work academic. It is a general comment on the need for social workers to be more vigilant, a comment on their competence. The considerable amount of direct quotes and a picture of Professor Stevenson at the press conference set up the inquiry report as an occasion for professional introspection. She is talking to the press and beyond them to the profession, the 'superaddressee' (Bakhtin 1986: 126). The details of professional failings are strong but can be heard as fair and typical of the everyday dilemmas of social work. Occurring in this context and with the report organised in this way, it might be seen as appropriate intra-professional scrutiny. Had similar comments been reported in the national press, they would be heard as 'hostile'.

While the report on page 5 may be introspective and cautioning, other parts of the *Community Care* coverage are far from apologetic. On the adjoining page 4 is a report of a study by the NSPCC which found a 35 per cent rise in the number of children on the child protection register. The two pieces are linked by an umbrella sub-headline, thereby making a strong connection between the specific case and the general situation:

Professionals fear more tragedies like Stephanie Fox as Child Abuse registers rocket.

Despite the headline, 'Staff increase needed to tackle rise in child abuse', the report on the NSPCC study does not suggest that there is more child abuse, but that social workers are better at identifying it. However, this increased vigilance requires more social workers to supervise the cases, with the Stephanie Fox seen as an example of the type of case that may happen again:

[. . .] (the inquiry report) confirms the view that the tragedy is in danger of being repeated because the rise in known cases continues to outpace over-stretched departments.

This is reported as a general situation and not related to Wandsworth's cuts. Just as the national press had transformed the case of Stephanie Fox from child murder to social work negligence and then into a political story and a critique of the poll tax, so the professional press transforms the story into a report about social workers getting better at identifying child abuse and the consequent need for more resources. It is not a case of social work failure, on the contrary, the profession is needed more than ever.

This theme of the need to enhance social work resources is developed further in the editorial 'Comment' on page 11 (see Appendix 2). The first paragraph concentrates on linking this case to the Maria Colwell case and re-visits the ongoing concerns about professional failings – closer cooperation, greater resources and more careful records. The rest of the Comment concentrates on the equation between cuts and abuse. It puts both sides of the argument as to whether child abuse is unaffected or exacerbated by cuts in services. Another voice is added to the case: the Prime Minister is quoted that Wandsworth has a 'good record'. The editor's answer to this dilemma is to recommend 'a bold experiment' to help resolve the issue:

> The experiment should begin by asking how much and what kind of resources are needed to reduce if not eradicate abuse. What would the nature of such a service be, how would it target its resources and how much would it cost?

In a climate of press coverage which has generally moved away from blaming social work failure to blaming cuts in services, the professional press is pushing the link further. It is more that good social work practice is able to identify and monitor child abuse. The NSPCC report had suggested that better social work activity had led to greater identification and the problem was one of resources to monitor these new cases. In a similar way, it is often debated whether more police increases or decreases reported crime – more police may detect more crime and hence increase the crime rate. Here, however, the opposite is being suggested: an increase in social work and related services can decrease and even eradicate child abuse. This must be the strongest claim yet for the centrality of social work to handling child abuse since it is suggested that the extent of social work and the extent of child abuse are linked directly. More social work might identify more child abuse, but even more social work might reduce it. The profession has transformed tragedy and criticism into a self-promotional discourse. Social work is not the problem but the solution.

Conclusion

The narrative of the murder of Stephanie Fox has been transformed by the national, local and professional press in a number of different ways and directions. It has moved through a depiction of the 'monster' of Stephen Fox, the 'incompetence' of social workers, the cuts in council services to criticisms of the poll tax, social work policies of placing them in protective custody and ambitions to eradicate child abuse through social work. This widespread direction of blames and claims clearly demonstrates that the death of a child can be used to posit a wide variety of interpretations. It is often difficult to establish a clear link between the nature of the interpretation and the socio-political ambitions of the mediators who interpret on behalf of readers.

The mainstay of this chapter has been with the nature of categorisation and accountability in media reporting. How do various commentators outside social work make claims using categorisation and developing versions of accountability? In ways similar to those we have observed in earlier chapters, there is the manipulation and rhetorical display of categories. What sort of case was Stephanie Fox? What sort of case was Victoria Climbié? The first was a child protection case, but it was not decided that this was a child rescue case (she should have been removed from her father). In the Climbié case, the contrast was between 'being in need' and 'being at risk'. In both cases, the main charge is a failure to adequately interpret information that was readily available. Both are post hoc formulations which have emerged in particular arenas which have highlighted extreme formulations of criticism, blame and accountability. As we have moved beyond the typical sites and contexts of everyday social work practice, we see how events can easily move from the routine to the spectacular. Working in conditions of extreme risk, are social workers prepared to continue in an atmosphere in which protective practice is always uppermost?

10 Conclusion

It might be expected that a book on social work would conclude with an overview of the current state of the profession and offer (usually upbeat) comments on proposed ways forward. In contrast, our approach to research has required us to be somewhat detached from the process of offering clear answers to straightforward questions concerning what social work is or should be. We have not looked at social work in terms of ethics or values, good practice or failures nor macro questions of policy or politics, important though these are. We have not considered social work as either liberating or alienating. Instead we suggested that important insights can be gained by concentrating on social work as a mundane, everyday activity; a job carried out in meetings, phone calls, case files and home visits, albeit one which often involves dilemmas, strong emotions and life-changing decisions. But then many human services workers face similar demands.

Neither have we been concerned with the communicative and interaction processes as ends in themselves, as might some language analysts. In essence we have focused on how language and interaction get used to enact certain activities and bring about, modify and maintain categorisations, and how this is done in ways which render these and social workers' actions accountable. We have shown these two to be important concepts across the key sites of social work, as professionals manage everyday demands and dilemmas – what sort of case is this? how do I display my practice as justifiable and competent? We see such practices as consequential for those involved and have considered how they are fed into debates already taking place within the profession. We have sought a dialogue between the researcher and the professional, concerned to find a balance between distanced analysis and involved professional reasoning. This is not straightforward, particularly when we have tried to comment on the practice implications of our research, a topic which researchers on language often avoid (see Silverman 1997: 212). Before we outline our suggestions in detail, we will briefly discuss on what basis we consider it is legitimate for discourse analysts to make such comments.

Neither evidence-based nor reflective practice

In the introduction, we outlined two major approaches to research in social work – evidence-based practice and reflective practice – and suggested that our approach would be different from both. Given our interest in the construction of character, it is worth asking what sort of character of the social worker is constructed by the different approaches and how ours differs.

Evidence-based practice comes with a rather mechanistic view of the social worker, which Schon (1983) describes as 'rational-technical'. The professional is expected to make a straightforward link between the attributes of a particular case and the generalities of research findings. As Webb (2001: 63) notes:

> Evidence-based practice assumes that rational agents (e.g. social workers) draw the obvious logical consequences of evidence-based findings, to apply fundamental logical principles about the likelihood of action achieving certain ends that respect the axioms of a behavioural probability calculus.

Research findings are seen as providing evidence of causal links between social and personal problems and the attributes of people or relationships. Furthermore it is assumed that research can identify specific interventions that 'work', enabling unproblematic connections between assessment and intervention. The professional merely has to identify the problems in a case and apply the appropriate intervention in order to achieve particular outcomes. A number of writers have criticised this view of rationality and proposed a more complex view of how social work gets done (for example: Parton 2000; Webb 2001; Witkin and Harrison 2001).

The reflective practitioner is a more rounded character. Practice decisions are seen as too complex to be based only on the implementation of research findings. Instead the professional is seen as responding to the local context of service delivery and the specific needs of a client, even when 'the evidence' is not necessarily available (Clarke and Proctor 1999: 979). The practitioner turns to intuition and tacit knowledge to assess situations and make decisions. As Schon (1983: 5) writes:

> Because the unique case falls outside the categories of existing theory and technique, the practitioner cannot treat it as an instrumental problem to be solved by applying one of the rules in her store of professional knowledge. The case is not 'in the book'. If she is to deal with it competently, she must do so by a kind of improvisation, inventing and testing in the situation strategies of her own devising.

Such a characterisation views the professional as actively searching for solutions to problems, drawing on experience and hunches rather than research findings. However such a view of practice still portrays the professional as standing outside everyday tasks and applying a linear model of assessment, analysis and decision-making, even if the 'theory' is based on experience. It implies that there is a form of analysis which is separate from, and more measured than, everyday formulations. However, as Ixer (1999: 519) notes, reflection is a 'social construction': all forms of analysis necessarily trade on processes which make up professional practices. In other words, what constitutes 'reflecting on practice' as well as 'reflection in practice' still depends on a wide range of contextual features: who is the audience, what forms of justification are preferred, how are versions produced jointly, what displays of competence are expected, etc. It might be suggested that the narratives of cases provided to the interviewer in Chapter 3 are reflections on practice.

Unearthing the 'seen but unnoticed'

Our approach has not been to attribute everyday practices to explanations which are seen in terms of applying theory to practice, whether evidence-based or experiential. Instead we view everyday social work practice as involving complex sets of language practices, with rhetorical devices and interactional moves deployed to manage communicative challenges in specific encounters. Our suggestion is that social workers (clients and other professionals) act in order to make assessments, display competence, persuade others, etc. This approach is exemplified in the concept of categorisation. Social workers would be expected (even required) by bureaucratic processes to categorise cases in terms of various types in order to direct their work – for instance, if the family problems are seen as caused by deficit parenting, then interventions should aim to promote parenting skills. For us, categorisation is much more pervasive; it is seen in terms of interactional, linguistic and rhetorical features and a constituent feature of all communication. Similarly, in everyday usage, accountability refers to processes which keep a check on the professional (e.g. the supervision session or the audit exercise). For us, however, accountability is implicit in social workers' explanations and it runs through everyday practice. It is essentially a distinction between outcome and process. For the social worker, defining the character of Kathy Malcolm in Chapter 4 was the aim of the case conference. Once categorised as a deficit parent, the appropriate intervention could be established. For us, however, the interest was in the unfolding process of categorisation during the case conference and this involved a complex set of interdependent interactional moves. As Giddens (1979: 43) says:

> A text is therefore not to be regarded as a 'fixed form' which is then somehow related *en bloc* to particular intentions; it should be studied as the concrete medium and outcome of a process of production, reflexively monitored by its author or reader.

Our characterisation of the social worker is therefore that of the interactional strategist, who strives to manage the succession of encounters which constitutes the professional world and who does so by deploying a range of linguistic and rhetorical skills. Such a character is strategic, artful and Machiavellian.

This strategic artfulness can come with various degrees and kinds of self-awareness. The complex skills and processes required to negotiate the social world is illustrated in Garfinkel's study of Agnes (1967: Chapter 5). Agnes was brought up as male until aged 17 but then began to dress and act as a woman and eventually had a sex change operation. During and after the operation, she had a series of conversations with the researcher about the work necessary to be a 'natural normal female'. What emerged was a complex range of behaviours and performances to avoid disclosure, as well as convincing those that knew her biography that she had been female all along. Heritage (1984: 182) describes her as a 'sensitive ethnographer of gender' as she deployed the skills and devices necessary to be female. These included learning details of presentation, behaviour and in particular her constructing and managing a 'missing' biography. She anticipated potentially difficult situations but also had to manage unexpected threats to discovery. As Garfinkel (1967: 184) notes, 'her devices were continually directed to, indeed, they consisted of a Machiavellian management of practical circumstances'. Far from being a clearly discernible and taken-for-granted category, a moral fact, Agnes was able to show the researcher that gender entails a vast range of performances.

Our suggestion has been that the social worker (but also clients and other professionals) is constantly deploying a range of skills, devices and methods to manage the encounters of social work. Unlike Agnes, many of these are so natural that they are 'seen but unnoticed' (Garfinkel 1967: 180). However in some encounters actors may be more aware of their use of such skills. For example the categorisation work about Kathy in the case conference in Chapter 4 suggests that each professional managed their contributions in such a way that they were paying particular attention to the categorisation work of others. In Chapter 7 Hilary James is also sensitive to the way she talks and acts in social work encounters, her 'being watched' by the social workers in the home visit or her being 'on trial' in the case conference. In Chapter 6, we saw that the case notes included particular depictions of the mother to construct her as an uncooperative client and to justify the removal of the children.

It is here that *reflexivity*, rather than reflection (Taylor and White 2000: 197), becomes an issue for all concerned – social workers, clients, other professionals, commentators, and researchers. Reflexivity is an important concept to the human sciences. In line with the discussion above, we will discuss it first as a feature of everyday life, relied upon by all actors, and as offering important insights in action and practice. In this sense, reflexivity refers to everyday activities by which members of a community monitor, react to and report on what is going on and treat it as normal and accountable. As Lynch (2000: 26–27) says 'it is an unavoidable feature of the way actions are performed, made sense of and incorporated into social settings [. . .] it is impossible to be unreflexive'. Macbeth (2001: 51, 52) provides a vignette of a classroom as a setting in which teacher and pupils 'assemble the order and structure of the lesson'. The children file into the room, sit down and the teacher starts to talk. The students continue to talk as the teacher asks a question about how a fraction can be described. Various students provide incorrect answers and the chatter continues. However the teacher then says:

> Who remembers a fraction that equals one half?
> (2.0) (the chatter declines)

Macbeth argues that at this point the various conversations between students cease and everyone accepts that the lesson has now started. Consequently certain conventions of questions/answers sequences, appropriate audience, etc. now apply.

The author suggests that various attempts by the teacher to engage the class had failed but by organising the question in terms of 'who remembers' rather than 'who can tell me', a previous version of the class is constructed and affiliation to an orderly lesson is sought:

> Reflexively, the choice (to stop talking) urges the children to become 'ordinary' students, unremarkably there and without nomination-relevant features, and even to hear the choice is to become implicated in the production of the normal order of the room.
>
> (2001: 54)

In this example we can see how managing everyday work situations trades on the skills and competences of being a teacher and being a pupil. It points to communication and affiliation processes which are 'seen but unnoticed' as well as learnt through routine role-governed practice. Such skills might be said to constitute 'tacit knowledge'.

This suggests that there may be a range of positions in relation to 'seen but unnoticed', which actors have different levels of explicit awareness of, and in view of which they pay less or more attention to the rhetorical and interactional skills. At one extreme is Agnes who is constantly and acutely aware of the skills required and performances necessary to be female. At the other extreme might be the reluctant children who gradually accept that the lesson has started. The link between reflexivity and making practice available for discussion is obvious. What is of specific interest for this project is where the researcher and the social worker fit in.

The balance between closeness and distance

To explore further the notion of 'seen but unnoticed' requires a balance between distance and closeness for both researcher and social worker. This is reflected in the ethnomethodologist's plight: on the one hand, s/he may be concerned to identify closely with the world of practitioners in order to analyse their everyday skills and competencies; on the other hand, s/he also wishes to refrain from making the kind of judgements which that world inevitably demands. Such a position may be questioned, since by taking on the members' world, the researcher is inevitably also taking on the evaluative positions that are embedded in the everyday practices. The challenge is thus to make those evaluations explicit for both the researcher and the professional. In this way researcher and practitioner face similar questions and suggestions for practice become central to the research process. This raises issues to do with where, when and how to comment on practice.

The researcher who comments on practice

As Hall *et al.* (2003b: 223) suggest, a more complex dialogue is needed between researcher and practitioner, 'making things more complicated' with research as only one of several voices which contribute to change. As Ortner (1999) points out, social science is nowadays both an agent in and an object of public culture (for instance, academics, novelists and media journalists constantly subsume one another in their efforts to tell 'the truth' about particular social or cultural realities or worlds: scientific results are quoted alongside experiential voices in media reports; social scientific studies comment on media representations of their topic of enquiry). Ortner (1999: 83) asks herself: as the voice of human sciences has become 'only one voice, one entry, within an enormously complex and multi-vocal universe of "public culture". In this context, what – if anything – is its distinctive contribution?' Particularly the chapters on media representations and public inquiry have high-lighted some of the ways in which public accountability can exercise strongly evaluative scrutiny. We do not wish to add to these strong, authoritative voices. In contrast, our specific contribution will aim to form alliances with the professionals. Hall *et al.* (2003b: 233ff.) summarise a variety of approaches to research which render things more complex, try to find positive ways to capture that complexity and hopefully lead to more thoughtful, sensitive and productive interventions. It may not direct social workers' decision-making, but seeks instead to illuminate the landscape for decision-makers, providing frames for thinking about it.

Thick description renders simplistic solutions superficial

As discourse research displays the contingent complexity of talk and interaction in social work encounters, it is crucial that a position is formulated that recognises that any changes to practice are equally complex, often with unintended conse-quences. For instance, the strict categorisation of and different priority given to 'family support', as opposed to 'child protection' cases, noted in Chapter 8 was presumably not the intention of the legislators of the Children Act 1989. A number of commentators on social work have expressed concern at the development of formal systems for regulating practice, often based on research findings (Parton 2003, Garrett 2003). As Jordon and Jordan (2000: 205) note:

> What [social work] does not need is the dreary, mechanistic, systematic, technocratic approach that puts clients into categories, and produces a ready-made package according to a pseudo-scientific classification of their deficits.

The danger is that findings from discourse research are also turned into rigid regulation. For example, it might be suggested that the way in which home visits are carried out is made more precise following the findings in Chapter 4 that there was vagueness about the purpose of the encounter. The Laming report (Laming 2003) made some suggestions about this. Similarly with the move to electronic case files discussed in Chapter 6 we note how recording may become more cautious. Consequently, particular procedures (or software) might be established which require the social worker to be more explicit about agreements made or expectations required. However, how such procedures are carried out will itself become part of the interactional task of the encounter: made more explicit if the interactional encounter requires it or backgrounded if this is preferred. For example Packman and

Hall (1998: 180ff.) note that meetings between professionals and families whose function was to plan services were sometimes used to bring to the attention of the client particular features which they had found hard to discuss in other situations, say hygiene or diet. Other criticisms were more commonly reserved for one-to-one sessions. In other words social workers are able to background or foreground formal procedures depending on interactional requirements.

A focus on interactional practices as accomplishments comes with a risk of admiring the artfulness of practice, implying a hesitation to recommend change. However, change is inevitably part of the landscape of professional practice and is determined as much by negotiation and compromise as by authority and evidence. We agree with Foucault (1981: 12) that change should be left to the dynamics of the ones nearest to the action to sort out what needs to be done, rather than reformers acting from above: 'the problem is one for the subject who acts'.

Our discussion has explored the notion of the social worker as uncertain of their professional authority and that there are advantages to promoting such uncertainty (Parton 1998). By stepping back from scientific approaches to social work, the 'humble accounts' (Lynch 1997: 371) of social workers and clients about complex and difficult situations open arenas for discussion and negotiation. For example, in Chapter 7 we noted how Hilary James resists attempts to categorise herself as a poor parent. These should be taken seriously in attempts to promote participation. However, institutional arrangements to build rigid and stigmatising formulations place constraints on such communication.

We do not privilege professional accounts, but nor do we suggest that their practices are necessarily alienating. Both social worker and clients have skills and competencies to manage encounters. Social workers manipulate legal and formal structures to control, clients have opportunities to resist. Policy and practice aimed at client participation continues to be developed. Whilst we have seen social workers more often in control of such encounters, as in the case conference (Chapter 3) or the home visit (Chapter 4), in other work it is less clear. Lloyd (1992: 121) for example investigates interrogative interviews in which children are encouraged to disclose sexual abuse. Although the questioning can be said to encourage such disclosure, the author is able to show examples of children who resist, concluding that coercive practice is far from settled.

In summary, changes in the nature of interaction between social workers, clients and other professionals are inevitable. However, attempts to regulate such changes through procedures and regulations will always take place against the backdrop of competing voices, positions and the contingent demands of everyday professional encounters.

Promoting a discourse analytical viewpoint for social work

There are a number of ways in which we feel that a discourse analytical approach can be outlined, discussed and extended. It is being suggested that the social work profession may gain from developing the skills and frameworks for examining the nature of talk and interaction. In this way their sensitivity to their own communication with clients and other professionals becomes an object for examination and discussion. Silverman (1997: 130) in particular has discussed the implications for practice of conversation analysis, suggesting that the focus should not be on 'communication problems' but looking at the functions of communication sequences. Sharing analysis on the basis of data transcripts and categories of discourse analysis offers one method for this. For example, by establishing a forum in which the social worker can be shown to be undermining the client's requests for a service of family therapy during the home visit analysed in Chapter 5, hidden processes in the decision-making could be brought out into the open. The importance of the detailed study of language and interaction is that it moves away from concentrating on social work theory to scrutiny of actual practice, for as Peräkylä (1995: 333) notes in a study of AIDS counsellors: 'the counsellors' own practice is even more sophisticated than their theory'.

There may be opportunities for a more general training programme in which discourse analysis becomes a feature of professional skills and competencies. Psathas (1990) suggests a number of directions for applied conversation analysis: to delineate the features of interaction, to compare them between settings and select particular competencies which are noted for education and training. In a similar vein, Tapsell (2000) concentrates on the deployment of narrative theory and analysis to improve the diet history-taking skills of trainee dieticians (e.g. alertness to narrative markers as a check on pace and direction). We suggest that these skills are often deployed by professionals unthinkingly and that there are advantages to making them visible and available for discussion, both to challenge and enhance practice.

Categorisation and accountability as a professional matter

While we suggest that social workers develop ways of broadening their views about communication with clients and other professionals, we are hesitant to see this as purely a problem for the individual worker. The categorisation and accountability practices which have been delineated in this study are so central to the everyday work of social workers that their discussion is required on a number of levels. As we have shown, the demands of categorisation and accountability permeate the dynamics of interactional sequence (for instance, in Chapter 7, because the client is categorised in the first encounter as having a drink problem, all the procedural processes set in motion referred back to that fact as a point of departure). Hence, there is a need to address categorisation and accountability in child protection work as a specific problem for discourse analytical research.

First, social workers put people into categories very easily. In Chapter 1 the social worker formed a view of the 'doting dad' within a few hours of contact. Whilst that formulation may have changed with later meetings it is also possible that the social worker added information which supported her initial picture. Munro (1996) has noted how versions of a case remain despite the emergence of disconfirming evidence. However the bureaucratic processes of child welfare often require definitive characterisation of clients to be established and confirmed in reports, assessments, diagnoses, etc. Once set on a particular path, a formulation becomes confirmed and tied into institutional inevitability. A particularly serious example of this was the way in which Victoria Climbié was seen, established and fixed, as discussed in Chapter 7. The question is: can practices be developed in ways which enable formulations to be tentative, uncertain and suspended?

Second, our research has shown how accountability is a routine dimension of all institutional interaction and an explicit requirement of certain situations. Chapter 4 in particular has shown that accountability is not just a matter of producing an account but all talk in the meeting also attends to the need to justify a version of the case, the client, etc. in front of specific audiences. The question to ask here is: can forms of practice be developed in which such strategic positioning no longer takes over the encounter and dominates its dynamics? Thorpe and Bilson (1998) have developed a model in which concerns and risks are shared between professionals, promoting instead the discretion to avoid child protection investigations by seeking positive alternatives. Whilst such approaches are unlikely to reduce displays of accountability, they may enable such accountability to be discussed and shared.

Third, as we saw in Chapter 4, the problem for professionals is not that they do not have similar meanings to terms, but terms become a part of the negotiation and argumentation processes of everyday professional and inter-professional practice. Furthermore, as we have shown in Chapter 8, hierarchies enter into this process, as seniority or the dominance of medical argumentation is often hard for social workers to counter. The point is perhaps not to be looking for a 'common language'; rather, engaging in debate about how people use terms like 'concern' as linked to categorisation, action and the allocation of resources.

Fourth, as we saw in Chapters 4 and 5, encounters between social workers, clients and other professionals like the case conference or home visit have multiple purposes. The different frames of reference and activity that apply may on occasion be at cross-purposes. Publicly and professionally voiced expectations that home visits must have a clear purpose need to be weighed against the demands of the situation of contact where a working relationship between children, social workers and families is central. In the case conference displays of agreement between professionals needs to be balanced with ways of exploring differences. Again this hints at the need for a setting in which agreement and difference can be discussed without undermining working relationships.

Fifth, in Chapters 6 and 8 we have drawn attention to the field of tension between, on the one hand, the ongoing private nature of case notes, constructed for local audiences and, on the other hand, their scrutiny during the public inquiry where case notes are used as a reliable and unproblematic basis for examining the actions of professionals. Professional alertness to and insight into the consequences of the re-use of notes on later occasions is one contribution which discourse analysis can offer. At the same time, current developments towards instant electronic sharing of case notes with other professionals, while seeking an enhancement of inter-agency information exchange, are likely to transform the very nature of note taking: more cautious and hesitant, concerned more with inter-agency accountability and stripped of the advantages which diary-like, written in-house notes once offered.

Sixth, the balance between discrediting categorisations and working with the client was discussed in Chapters 5 and 7. The issue of developing an ongoing working relationship with the client and constructing assessments of parent's failings has been long debated in social work. In some systems this has resulted in families having two social workers, one concerned with assessment and another with providing a service (Hood 1997). Our study suggests that, whatever the organisational arrangements, working with categorisations of clients is an inevitable feature of social work practice. However there may be approaches to working with families which do not require that categorisations necessarily direct the intervention.

Finally, in Chapters 8 and 9 we discussed the ways in which social work is from time to time thrust into the spotlight as high profile cases lead to widespread review and criticism. It is likely that the issues at stake in social work with children and families will remain ones which continue to cause controversy and public concern, as discussed in Chapter 9. Commentators continue to debate the significance of the recent high profile (and thorough) public inquiry, media coverage and legislative response, the Victoria Climbié Inquiry (Laming 2003). The long-term impact remains to be seen. Such an inquiry directs attention to the everyday processes at work in child welfare and how social workers (and other professionals) manage such dilemmas. Categorisation and accountability emerged as central issues, how the case was categorised one way rather than another and how professionals constructed accounts for their work, as we saw in Chapter 8. The topics of categorisation and accountability will thus remain of central focus and a discourse analytic approach can offer a major contribution to this debate.

Appendix 1

Transcriptions of data

The data in Chapters 3, 4, 5 and 7 represent talk between an interviewer and social worker, in a case conference, between a social worker and a client, and between an interviewer and a client, respectively. It is displayed without conventional punctuation so as not to impose a structure on the talk. Instead transcription conventions are used to signify pauses, emphasis and overlapping talk. These conventions are similar to those developed by Jefferson (in Atkinson and Heritage, 1984) but with some exceptions.

43 SW:	This is the social worker's turn of speech and the 43rd turn in these data, indicating how far into these data this extract occurs.
(.)	Short pause.
(3)	Longer pause with number of seconds indicated.
.	Point is used to break up longer stretches of text without implying a pause.
underline	Emphasis.
[SW: yes]	Backchannelling, comments that encourage the speaker to continue talking.
(inaudible)	Transcriber was unable to hear what was said.
(overlapping)	Speakers talk over one another.
(mother)	Role specified where the speaker uses a name.
(laughter)	Other comments by the transcriber.
w-	Word unfinished.

Chapter 6 displays case notes from social work files and Chapter 8 makes use of transcriptions from the Victoria Climbié Inquiry which uses conventional punctuation.

Appendix 2

Guardian
19 August 1989

Death of child in care sparks inquiry call
<name>, Social Services Correspondent

A Magistrate called yesterday for a full inquiry into how a child in the protection of social services was allegedly battered to death by her father after she and her two sisters had suffered a series of suspicious injuries.

The 22–year-old father, who has been charged with murder but cannot be named for legal reasons, was also involved in the accidental death of his first child.

Mr <name>, chairing the bench at Inner London Juvenile Court, said 'This is a disturbing, horrifying case involving the death of a child in care and I assume that at the end of it there is going to be a very penetrating inquiry into how it all came about.'

The court rejected an application by the man's partner that their younger daughters be returned to her or her parents rather than kept in the care of Wandsworth social services, south London, where they have been since the death of their sister two weeks ago.

Mrs <name>, acting as the children's guardian ad litem, opposed the application on grounds including the chance that the father, who is remanded in custody, might get bail.

The court heard that police were called to the family's council flat in the early hours of August 6 and found the elder child, aged almost three, with serious head injuries.

Police Inspector <name> said the father was threatening. Blood stains and human tissue were found in the toilet.

'The whole flat absolutely stank with excrement and urine,' said the inspector. The younger children's nappies did not appear to have been changed for 24 hours, he said.

They had been found in a small and dirty bedroom which they were apparently sharing with their sister.

'The children were lifeless, there was nothing in them. They didn't respond to kindness, to cuddles or laughing. Obviously they were in a state of shock.'

The 20-year old mother said that the flat had been clean and the children freshly changed when she had left the previous afternoon for an anniversary party at her parents' house. She returned at 5 am.

The court was told that the father's first child, a boy, had been the subject of a supervision order. He had choked in his vomit when apparently being fed and thrown in the air by his father. There had been no known police inquiry.

Injuries to the second child had been first reported in 1986, when she was two months old. She had been made subject of a care order as well as being placed, with the other children, on the at-risk register.

Mr <name>, the family's social worker since May, said he had recorded four incidents of bruising to the elder girl and one to each of the others. The mother said they were due to accidents, he said, and a doctor on one occasion substantiated this.

Mr <name> said he had not had much experience of such cases, but he had said this to his superiors.

Daily Mail
31 March 1990

Murdered girl was in danger all her life

By <name>, Chief Reporter

Little Stephanie Fox never had a chance. Her short, tragic life was one of continual misery. And when she was three she died at the hands of the drunken father she so feared amid the squalor he called home.

It happened despite the fact that she spent most of her life on a council's 'at risk' register, despite constant signs of physical and personal abuse noted by social workers and despite calls for increased vigilance after a series of child abuse scandals.

Last night, as father-of-five Stephen Fox, 23, was jailed for life at the Old Bailey for Stephanie's murder, Wandsworth social services in South London launched an urgent inquiry into why she was not taken into protective custody.

Fox, a caretaker, was high on drink and rock music when he literally shook and battered her to death. He showed no emotion as Mr Justice <name> told him: 'What you did must have filled everyone who saw and heard the case with horror.'

Scalded

It emerged last night that he regularly beat his daughter at their rubbish-strewn home at <name>, <estate>, Wandsworth where she slept in a broken jagged cot. She told social workers that her mother Alison also hit her.

Case workers knew that a son Fox had by Alison's sister choked to death in 1983 after he threw him into the air.

Private reports show that in December 1986, at four-and-a-half months, Stephanie was taken to hospital with burns to her neck and chin. Eighteen days later, social workers were told she had scalding on her thigh caused by an iron. She was put on the 'at risk' register.

The following March, bruises were found on her head and arm. Over the next three months more injuries were listed. A case conference noted: 'Alison was unable to care/cope with Stephanie.'

By June 1989 when she was almost three, the council was receiving calls from anxious neighbours. When social workers asked her about a bruise on her leg, Stephanie told them: 'I wouldn't eat my dinner and Daddy smacked me and threw me in the cot.'

They noted: 'She always looked sad and seemed to crave affection. She would always [unclear] everything.' One even wrote: 'Something made me frightened knowing Stephanie was alone with Stephen.' Days later that social worker was proved tragically right.

Her mother has since had another child. All three surviving children are in care awaiting adoption.

Wandsworth Borough News
6 April 1990

Inquiry launched into child's murder

Stephanie Fox was just three years old when she was finally killed by her drunken lout of a father.

In those three years she had been beaten, bruised, scalded and bitten. Her home, for the last year of her miserable life, was a filthy, squalid flat on the 19th floor of Wandsworth's <estate>.

If Wandsworth Social Services, the police, doctors, health visitors and NSPCC had not known of what was happening to Stephanie there would be justifiable outrage.

But they did know. And that makes it much, much worse.

For the officials charged with the protection of this little girl regularly visited her. They saw the bruises and the scald marks, they saw the filthy state of her home and they had full access to the medical records that testify to what happened, not once, but again and again and again.

They held case conferences and discussed how best they could help the family. Not once but again and again and again.

The fact is that Stephanie Fox died, horribly, while Wandsworth Social Services, the police and other agencies talked.

There is no doubt that these various agencies did their well-meaning best. Indeed worried Social Services staff went so far as to re-investigate the death of the first child to die at the hands of Stephen Fox in the light of injuries to Stephanie.

But they continued to follow fashionable and accepted dictat that a child is best off with his or her family. No matter what sort of a life that child is given.

Members of Stephanie's family told social workers and the NSPCC that the little girl was being beaten by Fox and her mother.

Undoubtedly those warnings figure in concerned reports by social workers. There will have been more case conferences. More talking.

Social workers chose to 'monitor the situation'. More talking.

The child had just one break. Just one chance. That came when she was taken from her family and placed in a foster home.

Suddenly there were no more unexplained bruises or bite marks. No more 'accidental' scald marks. Suddenly Stephanie stopped banging her head against walls – a classic sign of mental disturbance.

And once the bruises had faded, once the scalds and bites had healed. Once Stephanie had begun to put on the semblance of a normal, healthy toddler – she was returned to her family and it started again.

And last August three year old Stephanie Fox was murdered by her father in so violent a fashion that a woman just fainted when she saw the photographs.

Rightly, Wandsworth Council has commissioned an independent report which will seek to establish what lessons can be learned from Stephanie's murder.

We can put forward a few suggestions. We can suggest that social workers might not take incidents in isolation, particularly where there is a history of unexplained injuries to the child.

We can suggest that the 19th floor of a notoriously bleak tower block might not be the best possible environment for a child on the At Risk register. Indeed that the 19th floor of a tower block is an unsuitable environment for any family with small children.

We can suggest that if there is a dramatic improvement in the physical and mental condition of a child when she is in a foster home that there is a case for that child to remain in a place of safety, security and love.

And perhaps there is too much emphasis on retaining the accepted family unit at the expense of the interests of the child which must remain paramount.

Community Care
28 June 1990

Cuts contributed to child's death

By <name>

Financial cutbacks must take some of the blame for the death of three-year-old Stephanie Fox while she was on the Wandsworth child protection register, according to an independent inquiry report published last week.

Cash constraints in such areas as social work staffing levels, day nurseries and family support services are identified as contributing to the persistent physical abuse and eventual death of Stephanie last August.

The report is published at a particularly sensitive time for Wandsworth social services, with (trade union) claiming that the council plans to lop £5 million off the budget to keep the poll tax among the lowest in the country.

Social services committee chairwoman <name> denied that savings of £5 million were planned and pledged there would be no cuts in services.

The inquiry panel – chaired by Professor Olive Stephenson – also blamed the tragedy on poor communication between agencies and a tendency to underestimate Stephanie's plight.

In March Stephanie's father Stephen Fox, was sentenced to life imprisonment for murder, after the court heard that he had shaken his daughter to death following a heavy drinking session.

Stephanie was under a care order when she died but was staying with her parents.

Professor Stevenson told a press conference of her 'very grave concern' that the risk of such tragedies could only be increased by the appreciable number of children on child protection registers who had not been allocated social workers.

'In many London boroughs there are very serious problems of strategy and unallocated cases of child abuse which has to be a dangerous situation,' she said.

Wandsworth social services director <name> admitted that 'more than ten' child abuse victims were unallocated in the borough. He refused to confirm reports that social worker vacancy levels are running at 25 per cent.

A temporary failure of allocation in Stephanie's case is heavily criticised in the report. When the case was transferred between Wandsworth area offices four months before Stephanie's death there were no social work visits to the family for a month, during which time their health visitor was sick.

'We find it unacceptable that staffing levels should be such that there should be a lengthy delay in finding the new worker and handing over,' the report says.

The new social worker is criticised for his 'slowness in acting' on the case and in particular for failing to give sufficient weight to the views of Stephanie's day nursery.

Day nursery provision is also censured in the report. 'It is unacceptable that children . . . on the 'at risk' register should have to wait six months for a place or go to a nursery at a distance which places greater strain on parents and on the protection plan,' it says.

The shortage of places in day nurseries was largely caused by the council's money-saving policy of filling only two out of five staff vacancies, the report adds.

But Professor Stevenson was clear that Wandsworth health authority must also take a large share of the blame. There was no evidence which led inescapably to the view that Stephanie's death could have been predicted.

According to the report the SSD strove to maintain standards and were to a significant degree successful 'despite their financial restraint.'

Professor Stevenson highlighted four main points which emerged from the panel's 59 recommendations:

- Recruitment difficulties and financial pressures to hold down staffing levels weaken crucial interagency family support services;
- Separation of health and social services poses continuing problems for complex interagency child protection work;
- The need to keep a master record of all injuries to a child at risk;
- Professionals should recognise the significance of persistent parental denial of any responsibility for injuries to their children.

Community Care
28 June 1990

COMMENT

Action on child abuse

In April 1989 Stephanie Fox became a child abuse statistic. At three-years-old she had joined the sad and increasing roll call of children who have died as a result of physical and emotional abuse. Shaken to death as result of her father's heavy drinking bout, Stephanie's all too brief life has the awful familiarity of other child abuse tragedies (News, page 5). Reading the report, commissioned by the Wandsworth area child protection committee, it is impossible not to recall Maria Colwell. Her death, also investigated by Olive Stevenson, quickly gave short shrift to the then brave new world of generic social work departments. Many themes important to the Maria Colwell inquiry now re-surface with a sickening familiarity: the need for close inter-agency co-operation; the issue of resources; and the importance of keeping a careful record of all injuries.

Of particular significance in the Wandsworth report is the unambiguous reference to a failure of resources as one of the major contributory factors. That nursery places had been cut back, for example, was seen as crucial by the investigating panel. Further, (the trade union) has claimed that fieldwork vacancies in the borough stand at 25 per cent and that £5 million of cuts are planned in the current year (a claim denied by the chairperson of social services). At a local level this can be seen to support the critics of Wandsworth's policies who argue that evidence now exists for the relationship between very low poll tax and tragically poor levels of service. But the link between resources and child care tragedies goes much deeper. It is worth not-

ing two other recent events. First, recent statistics from the NSPCC, subsequently endorsed by the ADSS (The Association of Directors of Social Services), show that in the last year the number of children on registers, as a result of abuse, rose by 35 per cent. The NSPCC also estimated that 58,150 young people should have been on protection registers in England in 1989.

Second, Mrs Thatcher asserted in the Commons, following the Stephanie Fox review, that Wandsworth had a good record on 'social matters'. She said it had about 4 per cent more social workers in relation to its population than other inner London boroughs. Both claims indicate that the debate about the relationship between resources and the prevention of abuse to children is still being fought. Against those who argue that abuse is not related to levels of resources are those who maintain that child abuse is exacerbated by current cuts in services.

This debate prompts one relatively simple question: has the time come to involve one pilot area in a bold experiment that might help us resolve this issue? The experiment should begin by asking how much and what kind of resources are needed to reduce, if not eradicate abuse. What would the nature of such a service be, how would it target its resources and how much would it cost?

Such an experiment could never hope to be definitive and could be potentially embarrassing to any government prepared to reduce local government spending. But a carefully monitored project, in a multiracial inner city area with high indicators of social need, might help to resolve the connection between resources, good services and prevention. A project along these lines might take Stephanie Fox's death less tragically futile. The alternative seems to be yet more tragedies and more public debates about how paucity of resources helps or hinders.

Notes

2 Categorisation and accountability in professional texts and talk

1 Admittedly in recent years, the blameworthiness of patients for their illness has entered debates about policy and finance of health services (smoking, drugs, obesity, etc.) and what might be called 'surveillance medicine' (Armstrong 1995).
2 Child abuse as a socially constructed phenomenon has been suggested by a UK government report (Department of Health 1995: 15).

3 Collegial communication in policy review interviews

1 In recent years, policy review and audit in public services has taken on a variety of forms: 'quality assurance', 'inspection teams', 'performance monitoring', etc., each emphasising the inspectorial nature of such exercises.
2 Pithouse and Atkinson (1988) engage in a similar discussion about the management of a category. In the case they analyse 'incest' is hinted at but never clearly attributed or defined.
3 Someone convicted under 'schedule 1' of the Children and Young Person's Act 1933 of an offence against children, which remains on a person's criminal record for life.
4 Please see Appendix 1 for information of the Transcription of data.

4 Inter-professional decision-making in a case conference

1 The meetings discussed in this chapter are more formal than those investigated by Boden (1995) or Housley (2000), being required by policy or procedure. They usually involve 'outsiders', clients and professionals from other agencies. 'In-house' meetings in social work are studied by White (1999).
2 Being on the child protection register means the child is considered to be 'at risk of significant harm', and this concern is made known to all appropriate professionals. A child protection plan sets out various interventions and if improvements occur the child's name can be removed from the register at a child protection review.
3 In one case conference observed, the psychotherapist said nothing for the first half of the meeting, but then made the definitive assessment which drew on the earlier discussion and became the agenda for the rest of the meeting.
4 Child Guidance units are now called Child and Adolescent Mental Health teams (CAMH).
5 The term 'grave concern' is used to define a category of child abuse and was still being used when the data was recorded. Therefore, to use those words implied legal consequences.
6 It is likely that the search for further assessment was motivated by the evidence required for case proceedings, as highlighted by the solicitor at an earlier meeting.

6 Reporting events in case notes

1 The analysis will only consider the running sheet of events and actions and not summary reports which assess or evaluate the overall state of affairs in the family or required interventions (e.g. reports to courts, core assessments, etc.).

7 Parents' accounts of social work

1 'Voluntary care' refers to children being placed in foster or children's homes without changing their parental status and hence not requiring a court order. Under the 1989 Children Act, this is termed 'offering accommodation'. However, the term 'voluntary care' has remained in use.

8 Justifying action in a public enquiry

1 As we are using the official transcripts of the inquiry, our data is also constituted differently from the transcripts in earlier chapters which have been specifically designed for discourse-analytical purposes.
2 The page and line numbers in the excerpts below are as used in the official transcript (see http://www.victoria-Climbie-inquiry.org.uk).
3 NAI = non-accidental injury.
4 Mrs Kouao also used 'Anna' for Victoria.

9 Narrative transformation in media reporting

1 'Gerrymandering' is the proverbial way of referring to a method of arranging election districts to the advantage of the political parties making the arrangement. The term was coined after Elbridge Gerry, Governor of Massachusetts, had district boundaries re-drawn for the Senate elections of 1812. The map of the state that he created had the shape of a salamander.
2 The 'poll tax' was a new approach to local taxation which attempted to link tax rates to local authority expenditure on services. It was called the 'poll tax' because it was based on residency rather than property and electoral lists were used as a basis for registration. The tax proved very controversial and was repealed a year later.
3 Aldridge (1994: 65) uses the coverage in the *Sun* to caution against a too mechanistic conception of the editorial process, since at the time it was supporting the Conservative government.

Bibliography

Adelsward, V. and Nilholm, C. (2000) 'Who is Cindy? Aspects of identity work in a teacher-parent-pupil talk in the special school', *Text*, 20(4): 545–568.

Aldridge, M. (1994) *Making Social Work News*, London: Routledge.

—— (1999) 'Poor relations: state social work and the press in the UK', in B. Franklin (ed.) *Social Policy, the Media and Misrepresentation*, London: Routledge.

Antaki, C. and Widdicombe, S. (eds) (1998) *Identities in Talk*, London: Sage.

Armstrong, D. (1995) 'The rise of surveillance medicine', *Sociology of Health and Illness*, 17(3): 393–404.

Aronsson, K. (1998) 'Identity-in-interaction and social choreography', *Research on Language and Social Interaction*, 31: 75–89.

Artinian, N.T., Lange, M.P., Templin, T.N., Stallwood, L.G. and Hermann, C.E. (2003) 'Functional health literacy in an urban primary care clinic', *The Internet Journal of Advanced Nursing Practice*, 5(2).

Atkinson, J.M. and Drew, P. (1979) *Order in Court*, London: Macmillan.

Atkinson, J.M. and Heritage, J. (eds) (1984) Structure of Social Action, Cambridge: Cambridge University Press.

Atkinson, P. (2004) 'The discursive construction of competence and responsibility in medical collegial talk', *Communication and Medicine*, 1(1): 13–23.

Bakhtin, M.M. (1981) *The Dialogic Imagination*, Austin: University of Texas Press.

—— (1984) *Problems in Dostoevsky's Poetics*, ed. and trans. by Caryl Emerson, Manchester: Manchester University Press.

—— (1986) *Speech Genres and Other Late Essays*, Austin: University of Texas Press.

Baldock, J. and Prior, D. (1981) 'Social workers talking to clients: a study of verbal behaviour', *British Journal of Social Work*, 11: 19–38.

Barrett, R. (1996) *The Psychiatric Team and the Social Definition of Schizophrenia*, Cambridge: Cambridge University Press.

Barthes, R. (1975) *S/Z*, London: Jonathan Cape.

Bauman, R, and Briggs, C.L. (1990) 'Poetics and performance: critical perspectives on language and social life', *Annual Review of Anthropology*, 19: 59–88.

Baynham, M. and Slembrouck, S. (1999) 'Speech representation and institutional discourse', *Text*, 19: 439–458.

Beck, U. (1992) [1986] *Risk Society: Towards a New Modernity*, trans. by Mark Ritter, and with an introduction by Scott Lash and Brian Wynne, London: Sage.

Bell, A. (1991) *The Language of News Media*, Oxford: Blackwell.

—— (1996) 'An account of the experience of 51 families involved in child protection conferences', *Child and Family Social Work*, 1: 43–55.

—— (1999) 'Working in partnership in child protection', *British Journal of Social Work*, 29(3): 437–455.

Bergmann, J.R. (1992) 'Veiled moralities: notes on discretion in psychiatry', in P. Drew and J. Heritage (eds) *Talk at Work: Interaction in Institutional Settings*, Cambridge: Cambridge University Press.

Billig, M. (1985) 'Prejudice, categorization and particularisation: from a perceptual to a rhetorical approach', *European Journal of Social Psychology*, 15: 79–103.

—— (1987) *Arguing and Thinking: A Rhetorical Approach to Social Psychology*, Cambridge: Cambridge University Press.

—— (1999) 'Whose terms? Whose ordinariness? Rhetoric and ideology in Conversation Analysis', *Discourse and Society*, 10: 543–558.

Boden, D. (1995) 'Agendas and arrangements: everyday negotiations in meetings', in A. Firth (ed.) *The Discourse of Language in the Workplace*, Oxford: Pergamon.

Bourdieu, P. (1977) 'The economics of linguistic exchanges', *Social Science Information*, 16: 645–668.

Callon, M. (1986) 'Some elements of a sociology of translation: domestication of the scallops and the fishermen of St Brieuc Bay', in. J. Law (ed.) *Power, Action and Belief: A New Sociology of Knowledge*, London: Routledge.

Chatman, S. (1978) *Story and Discourse: Narrative Structure in Fiction and Film*, Ithaca: Cornell University Press.

Cicourel, A. (1974) 'Police practices and official records', in R. Turner (ed.) *Ethnomethodology*, Harmondsworth: Penguin.

—— (1976) *The Social Organisation of Juvenile Justice*, London: Heinemann.

—— (1983) 'Hearing is not believing: language and the structure of belief in medical communication', in S. Fisher and A. Todd (eds) *The Social Organisation of Doctor–Patient Communication*, Washington, DC: Center for Applied Linguistics.

Clarke, C and Proctor, S (1999) 'Practice development: ambiguity in research and practice', *Journal of Advanced Nursing*, 30(4): 975–982.

Cleaver, H. and Freeman, P. (1995) *Parental Perspectives in Cases of Suspected Child Abuse*, London: HMSO.

Cockcroft, R. and Cockcroft, S. (1992) *Persuading People: An Introduction to Rhetoric*, Basingstoke: Macmillan.

Collins, J. and Slembrouck, S. (2004) *You Don't Know What They Translate: Language Contact, Institutional Procedure, and Literacy Practice in Neighbourhood Health Clinics in Urban Flanders*, Gent: LPI Working Papers no. 19.

Corby, B., Millar, M. and Young, L. (1996) 'Parental participation in child protection work: rethinking the rhetoric', *British Journal of Social Work*, 24(4): 475–492.

Corby, B., Doig, A. and Roberts, V. (2001) *Public Inquiries into Abuse of Children in Residential Care*, London: Jessica Kingsley Publishers.

Cotterill, J. (2003) *Language and Power in Court: A Linguistic Analysis of the O.J. Simpson Trial*, Basingstoke: Palgrave Macmillan.

Coulthard, M. (1977) *An Introduction to Discourse Analysis*, London: Longman.

—— (1996) 'The official version: audience manipulation in police records of interviews with suspects', in C.R. Caldas-Coulthard and M. Coulthard (eds) *Texts and Practices: Readings in Critical Discourse Analysis*, London: Routledge.

Coupland, J., Robinson, J. and Coupland, N. (1994) 'Frame negotiation in doctor–elderly patient consultations', *Discourse and Society*, 5(1): 89–124.

Cuff, E.C. (1980) *Some Issues in Studying the Problem of Versions in Everyday Situations*, Manchester: Manchester University Occasional Papers no. 3.

Department of Health (1995) *Child Protection: Messages from Research*, London: HMSO.

Department of Health, Home Office and National Assembly of Wales (2001) *A Framework for the Assessment of Children in Need and Their Families*, London: Stationery Office.

Dingwall, R. (1977) '"Atrocity stories" and professional relationships', *Sociology of Work and Occupations*, 4: 371–396.

Dingwall, R. and Murray, T. (1983) 'Categorisation in accident departments: "good" patients, "bad" patients and "children"', *Sociology of Health and Illness* 5(2): 128–148.

Dingwall, R., Eekelaar, J, and Murray, T. (1983) *The Protection of Children: State Intervention and Family Life*, Oxford: Basil Blackwell.

Donzelot, J. (1980) *The Policing of Families: Welfare versus the State*, London: Hutchinson.

Douglas, M. (1992) *Risk and Blame: Essays in Cultural Theory*, London: Routledge.

Drew, P. (1990) 'Strategies in the Contest between Lawyer and Witness in Cross-Examination', in J. Levi and A. Walker (eds) *Language in the Judicial Process*, London: Plenum Press.

—— (1992) 'Contest evidence in courtroom cross-examination', in P. Drew and J. Heritage (eds) *Talk at Work: Interaction in Institutional Settings*, Cambridge: Cambridge University Press.

Edwards, D. (1991) 'Categories are for talking: on the cognitive and discursive bases of categorization', *Theory and Psychology*, 1(4): 515–542.

—— (1994) 'Script formulations: a study of event descriptions in conversations', *Journal of Language and Social Psychology*, 13 (3): 211–247.

—— (1997) *Discourse and Cognition*, London: Sage.

Ehrlich, S. (2002) 'Legal institutions, nonspeaking recipiency and participants' orientations', *Discourse and Society*, 13(6): 731–747.

Emerson, R.M. (1987) 'On last resorts', *American Journal of Sociology*, 87(1): 1–22.

Fairclough, N. (1991) *Discourse and Social Change*, Cambridge: Polity Press.

Farmer, E. and Owen, M. (1995) *Child Protection Practice: Private Risks and Public Remedies: Decision-making, Intervention and Outcome in Child Protection*, London: HMSO.

Floersch, J. (2002) *Meds, Money and Manners: The Case Management of Severe Mental Illness*, New York: Columbia University Press.

—— (2004) 'A method of investigating practitioner use of theory in practice', *Qualitative Social Work*, 3(2): 161–177.

Foucault, M. (1981) 'Questions of method: an interview', *Ideology and Consciousness*, 8: 3–14.

Fox Harding, L. (1997) *Perspectives in Child Care Policy*, London: Longman.

Franklin, B. (1998) *Hard Pressed: National Newspaper Reporting of Social Work and Social Services*, London: Reed Business Publications.

Franklin, B. and Parton, N. (2001) 'Press-ganged media reporting of social work and child abuse', in M. May, R. Page and E. Brunsdon (eds) *Understanding Social Problems: Issues in Social Policy*, Oxford: Blackwell.

Garfinkel, H. (1967) *Studies in Ethnomethodology*, Cambridge: Polity Press.

Garrett, P.M. (2003) 'Swimming with dolphins: the assessment framework, New Labour and new tools for social work with children and families', *British Journal of Social Work*, 33: 441–463.

Gergen, K. (1999) *An Invitation to Social Construction*, London: Sage.

Gibbons, J. (2003) *Forsenic Linguistics: An Introduction to Language in the Justice System*, Oxford: Blackwell.

Giddens, A. (1979) *Central Problems in Social Theory: Action Structure and Contradiction in Social Analysis*, London: Macmillan.

Gilbert, N. and Mulkay, M. (1984) *Opening Pandora's Box: A Sociological Analysis of Scientists' Discourse*, Cambridge: Cambridge University Press.

Gill, R., Potter, J. and Webb, A. (1991) 'Public policy and discourse analysis; a rhetorical approach', unpublished manuscript, Department of Human Sciences, Brunel University.

Gill, V.T. and Maynard, D.W. (1995) 'On "Labeling" in Actual Interaction: Delivering and Receiving Diagnoses of Developmental Delay', *Social Problems*, 42(1): 11–37.

Gilmore, A. (1988) *Innocent Victims*, London: Michael Joseph.

Goffman, E. (1968) [1961] *Asylums: Essays on the Social Situation of Mental Patients and Other Inmates*, Harmondsworth: Penguin.

—— (1974) *Frame Analysis: An Essay on the Organisation of Experience*, New York: Harper and Row.

—— (1981) *Forms of Talk*, Philadelphia: University of Pennsylvania Press.

—— (1983) 'The interaction order', *American Sociological Review*, 48: 1–17.

—— (1990) *Stigma: Notes on the Management of Spoiled Identity*, London: Penguin.

Goodwin, C. (1994) 'Professional vision', *American Anthropologist*, 96(3): 606–633.

Grice, H.P. (1975) 'Logic and conversation', in P. Cole and J.L. Morgan (eds) *Syntax and Semantics Volume 3: Speech Acts*, New York: Academic Press.

Gunnarsson, B., Linell, P and Nordberg, B. (1997) 'Introduction' in B. Gunnarsson, P. Linell and B. Nordberg (eds.) *The Construction of Professional Discourse*, Longman: Harlow.

Hak, T. (1989) 'Constructing a psychiatric case', in B. Torode (ed.) *Text and Talk in Social Practice*, Dordrecht: Foris.

—— (1992) 'Psychiatric records as transformations of other texts', in G. Watson and R.M. Seiler (eds) *Text in Context: Contributions to Ethnomethodology*, Newbury Park, CA: Sage.

Hall, C. (1997) *Social Work as Narrative: Storytelling and Persuasion in Professional Texts*, Aldershot: Ashgate.

Hall, C. and Slembrouck, S. (2001) 'Parent participation in social work meetings: the case of child protection conferences', *European Journal of Social Work*, 4(2): 143–160.

Hall, C., Juhila, K., Parton., N. and Pösö, T. (eds) (2003a) *Constructing Clienthood in Social Work and Human Services: Interaction, Identities and Practices*, London: Jessica Kingsley Publishing.

Hall, C., Parton, N., Juhila, K. and Pösö, T. (2003b) 'Conclusion: yes, but is this of any use?', in C. Hall, K. Juhila, N. Parton, and T. Pösö (eds) *Constructing Clienthood in Social Work and Human Services: Interaction, Identities and Practices*, London: Jessica Kingsley Publishing.

Hall, C., Sarangi, S. and Slembrouck, S. (1997a) 'Moral construction in social work discourse', in B. Gunnarsson, P. Linell and B. Nordberg (eds) *The Construction of Professional Discourse*, London: Longman.

—— (1997b) 'Silent and silenced voices: interactional construction of audience in social work talk', in A. Jaworski (ed.) *Silence: Interdisciplinary Perspectives*, Berlin: Mouton de Gruyter.

—— (1999a) 'Speech representation and the categorisation of the client in social work discourse', *Text*, 19(4): 539–570.

—— (1999b) 'The legitimation of the client and the profession in social work discourse', in S. Sarangi and C. Roberts (eds) *Talk, Work and the Institutional Order*, Berlin: Mouton de Gruyter.

Hallett, C. and Stevenson, O. (1980) *Child Abuse: Aspects of Interprofessional Cooperation*, London: Allen and Unwin.

Hardstone, G., Hartswood, M., Proctor, R., Slack, R., Voss, A. and Rees, G. (2004) 'Supporting informality: team working and integrated care records', paper presented at Computer Supported Cooperative Work Conference, Chicago, November.

Harré, R. (1985) 'Situational rhetoric and self-presentation', in J.P. Forgas (ed.) *Language and Social Situations*, New York: Springer-Verlag.

Harris, S. (2001) 'Fragmented narratives and multiple tellers: witness and defendant accounts in trials', *Discourse Studies*, 3(1): 53–74.

Have, P. ten (1991) 'Talk and interaction: a reconsideration of the "asymmetry" of doctor–patient interaction', in D. Boden and D.H. Zimmerman (eds.) *Talk and Social Structure: Studies in Ethnomethodology and Conversation Analysis*, Cambridge: Polity Press.

Hayes, D. and Devaney, J. (2004) 'Accessing social work case files for research purposes', *Qualitative Social Work*, 3(3): 313–333.

Heath, C. and Hindmarsh, J. (2002) 'Analysing interaction: video, ethnography and situated conduct', in T. May (ed.) *Qualitative Research in Action*, London: Sage

Her Majesty's Government (2003) *Every Child Matters*, Cmnd 5860, London: Stationery Office.

Heritage, J. (1984) *Garfinkel and Ethnomethodology*, Cambridge: Polity Press.

Heritage, J. and Sefi, S. (1992) 'Dilemmas of advice: aspects of the delivery and reception of advice in interactions between health visitors and first time mother', in P. Drew and J. Heritage (eds) *Talk at Work: Interaction in Institutional Settings*, Cambridge: Cambridge University Press.

Hester, S. (1998) 'Describing "Deviance" in School: Recognizably Educational Psychological Problems', in C. Antaki and S. Widdicombe (eds) *Identities in Talk*, London: Sage.

Hester, S. and Eglin, P. (eds) (1997) *Culture in Action: Studies in Membership Categorization Analysis*, Lanham, MD: International Institute for Ethnomethodology and Conversation Analysis and University Press of America.

Hills, A. (1980) 'How the press sees you', *Social Work Today*, 20 May: 19–20.

Holland, S. (1999) 'Discourses of decision making in child protection: conducting comprehensive assessments in Britain', *International Journal of Social Welfare*, 8: 277–287.

Holstein, J. and Miller, G. (eds) (1993) *Reconsidering Social Constructionism: Debates in Social Problems Theory*, New York: Aldine de Gruyter.

Home Office (2004) *Crime in England and Wales 2002/3*, London: Stationery Office.

Hood, S. (1997) 'Purchaser–provider separation in child and family social work: implications for service delivery and for the role of the social worker', *Child and Family Social Work*, 2: 25–35.

Housley, W. (2000) 'Story, narrative and team work', *The Sociological Review*, 48(3): 425–443.

Howarth, V. (1991) 'Social work and the media: pitfalls and possibilities', in B. Franklin and N. Parton (eds) *Social Work, the Media and Public Relations*, London: Routledge.

Hughes, E.C. (1958) *Men at Their Work*, Glencoe: Free Press.

Hyden, M. and Overlien, C. (2005) 'Applying narrative analysis to the process of confirming or disregarding cases of suspected sexual abuse', *Child and Family Social Work*, 10: 57–65.

Hymes, D. (1975) 'Breakthrough into performance', in D. Ben-Amos and K. Goldstein (eds) *Folklore: Performance and Communication*, The Hague: Mouton.

Ixer, G. (1999) 'There's no such thing as reflection', *British Journal of Social Work*, 29: 513–527.

Janis, I. (1982) *Groupthink*, Boston: Houghton Mifflin.

Jefferson, G. (1990) 'List construction as a task and resource', in G. Psathas (ed.) *Interaction Competence*, Washington: University of America Press.

Jefferson, G. and Lee, J. (1992) 'The rejection of advice: managing the problematic convergence of a "troubles-telling" and a "service encounter"', in P. Drew and J. Heritage (eds.) *Talk at Work: Interaction in Institutional Settings*, Cambridge: Cambridge University Press.

Jenkins, R. (2000) 'Categorization: identities, social process and epistemology', *Current Sociology*, 48: 7–25.

Johnson, S. (2004) 'Someone to watch over me'. Online. Available: http://www.open2.net/someonetowatch/about.html (accessed 25 April 2005).

Jokinen, A., Juhila, K. and Pösö, T. (1999) *Constructing Social Work Practices*, Aldershot: Ashgate.

Jonsson, L. and Linell, P. (1991) 'Story generations: from dialogical interviews to written reports in police interrogations', *Text*, 11(3): 419–440.

Jordan, B. with Jordan, C. (2000) *Social Work and the Third Way: Tough Love as Social Policy*, London: Sage.

Kagle, J.D. (1993) 'Record keeping: directions for the 1990s', *Social Work*, 38: 190–196.

Kent Child Protection Committee (2005) 'Policy and procedure for responding to children in need'. Online. Available: http://www.kcpc.org.uk/text.htm#sect3 (accessed 24 April 2005).

Kitzinger, J. (1996) 'Media representations of sexual abuse risks', *Child Abuse Review*, 5: 319–333.

—— (2000) 'Media templates: patterns of association and the (re)construction of meaning over time', *Media, Culture and Society*, 22(1): 64–84.

Kitzinger, J. and Skidmore, P. (1995) 'Playing safe: media coverage of child sexual abuse prevention strategies', *Child Abuse Review*, 4: 47–56.

Labov, W. (1972) *Language in the Inner City: Studies in Black English Venacular*, Philadelphia: Philadelphia University Press.

Labov, W. and Waletzky, J. (1967) 'Narrative analysis: oral versions of personal experience', in J. Helms (ed.) *Essays in the Verbal and Visual Arts*, Seattle: University of Washington Press.

Lakoff, G. (1987) *Women, Fire, and Dangerous Things: What Categories Reveal about the Mind*, Chicago: University of Chicago Press.

Laming, H. (2001) Preliminary Meeting of Victoria Climbié Inquiry 31 May 2001, Online. Available: http://www.victoria-climbie-inquiry.org.uk (accessed 19 April 2005).

—— (2003) *The Victoria Climbié Inquiry*, London: Stationery Office.

Latour, B. (1987) *Science in Action*, Milton Keynes: Open University Press.

Lave, J. and Wenger, E. (1991) *Situated Learning: Legitimate Peripheral Participation*, Cambridge: Cambridge University Press.

Lepper, G. (2000) *Categories in Text and Talk*, London: Sage.

Leudar, I. (1995) 'Reporting political arguments', in F.H. van Eemergen, R. Grootendorst, A. Blair and C.A. Willard (eds) *Reconstruction and application*, Proceedings of the Third Conference of ISSA, Amsterdam: Sic Sat.

Leudar, I and Antaki, C. (1996) 'Discourse participation, reported speech and research practices in social psychology', *Theory and Psychology*, 6: 5–29.

Linell, P. and Sarangi, S. (eds) (1998) 'Discourse across professional boundaries', special edition of *Text*, 18(2): 143–218.

Little, M., Madge, J., Mount, K., Ryan, M. and Tunnard, J. (2001) *Matching Needs and Services*, Dartington Academic Press, Dartington.

Lloyd, R. (1992) 'Negotiating child sexual abuse: the interactional character of investigative practices', *Social Problems*, 19(1): 109–124.

Locke, A. and Edwards, D. (2003) 'Bill and Monica: memory, emotion and normativity in Clinton's Grand Jury testimony', *British Journal of Social Psychology*, 42: 239–256.

Lynch, M. (1997) 'Ethnomethology without indifference', *Human Studies*, 20: 371–376.

—— (2000) 'Against reflexivity as an academic virtue and Source of Knowledge', *Theory, Culture and Society*, 17(3): 26–54.

Lynch, M. and Bogen, D. (1996) *The Spectacle of History: Speech, Text and Memory at the Iran–Contra Hearings*, Durham: Duke University Press.

Macbeth, D. (2001) 'On "reflexivity" in qualitative research: two readings, and a third', *Qualitative Inquiry*, 7: 35–68.

Maitland, K. and Wilson, J. (1987) 'Pronominal selection and ideological conflict', *Journal of Pragmatics*, 11(4): 495–512.

Mäkitalo, Ä. (2003) 'Accounting practices as situated knowing: dilemmas and dynamics in institutional categorisation', *Discourse Studies*, 5(4): 495–516.

Mäkitalo, Ä. and Säljö, R. (2002) 'Invisible people: institutional reasoning and reflexivity in the production of services and "Social Facts" in public employment agencies', *Mind, Culture and Activity*, 9(3): 160–178.

Manning, P. (1986) 'Texts as organisational echoes', *Human Studies*, 9: 287–302.

Margolin, L. (1997) *Under the Cover of Kindness: The Invention of Social Work*, Charlottesville, VA: University of Virginia Press.

Mehan, H. (1983) 'The role of language and the language of role in institutional decision making', *Language in Society*, 12: 187–211.

—— (1996) 'Beneath the skin and between the ears: a case study in the politics of presentation', in S. Chaiklin and J. Lave (eds) *Understanding Practice: Perspectives on Activity and Context*, Cambridge: Cambridge University Press.

—— (1997) 'The discourse of the illegal immigration debate: a case study in the politics of representation', *Discourse and Society*, 8: 249–270.

de Montigny, G. (1995) *Social Working: An Ethnography of Front-Line Practice*, Toronto: University of Toronto Press.

Munro, E. (1996) 'Avoidable and unavoidable mistakes in child protection work', *British Journal of Social Work*, 26: 793–808.

Nelson, B. (1984) *Making an Issue of Child Abuse: Political Agenda Setting for Social Problems*, Chicago: University of Chicago Press.

Nijnatten, C. van, Hoogsteder, M. and Suurmond, J. (2001) 'Communication in care and control: institutional interactions between family supervisors and parents', *British Journal of Social Work*, 31: 705–720.

Ochs, E. and Capps, L. (2001) *Living Narrative: Creating Lives in Everyday Storytelling*, Cambridge, MA: Harvard University Press.

Ortner, S. (1999) 'Generation X: anthropology in a media-saturated world', in G.E. Marcus (ed.) *Critical Anthropology Now: Unexpected Contexts, Shifting Constituencies, Changing Agendas*, Santa Fe: SAR Press.

Packman, J. and Hall, C. (1998) *From Care to Accommodation: Support, Protection and Control in Child Care Services*, London: Stationery Office.

Parton, N. (1991) *Governing the Family: Child Care, Child Protection and the State*, Basingstoke: Macmillan.

—— (1998) 'Risk, advanced liberalism and child welfare: the need to rediscover uncertainty and ambiguity', *British Journal of Social Work*, 28: 5–27.

—— (2000) 'Some thoughts on the relationship between theory and practice in and for social work', *British Journal of Social Work*, 30: 449–463.

—— (2003) 'Rethinking professional practice: the contributions of social constructionism and the feminist "Ethic of Care"', *British Journal of Social Work*, 33: 1–16.

—— (2004) 'From Maria Colwell to Victoria Climbié', *Child Abuse Review*, 13: 80–94.

Parton, N. and O'Byrne (2000) *Constructive Social Work: Towards a New Practice*, London: Macmillan.

Parton, N., Thorpe, D. and Wattam, C. (1997) *Child Protection: Risk and the Moral Order*, Basingstoke: Macmillan.

Peräkylä, A. (1995) *AIDS Counselling: Institutional Interaction and Clinical Practice*, Cambridge: Cambridge University Press.

Pettinari, C.J. (1988) *Task, Talk, and Text in the Operating Room: A Study in Medical Discourse*, Norwood, NJ: Ablex.

Pithouse, A. (1987) *Social Work: The Organisation of an Invisible Trade*, Aldershot: Gower.

Pithouse, A. and Atkinson, P. (1988) 'Telling the case: occupational narrative in a social work office', in N. Coupland (ed.) *Styles of Discourse*, London: Croom Helm.

Potter, J. and Reicher, S. (1987) 'Discourse of community and conflict: the organisation of social categories in accounts of a "riot"', *British Journal of Social Psychology*, 26: 25–40.

Potter, J. and Wetherell, M. (1987) *Discourse and Social Psychology: Beyond Attitudes and Behaviour*, London: Sage.

Prince, K. (1996) *Boring Records?: Communication, Speech and Writing in Social Work*, London: Jessica Kingsley.

Prior, L. (2003) *Using Documents in Social Research*, London: Sage.

Psathas (1990) 'Introduction: methodological issues and recent developments in the study of naturally occurring interaction', in G. Psathas (ed.) *Interactional Competence*, Washington: University of America Press.

Raffel, S. (1979) *Matters of Fact: A Sociological Inquiry*, London: Routledge & Kegan Paul.

Ravotas, D. and Berkenkotter, C. (1998) 'Voice in the text: the uses of reported speech in a psychotherapist's notes and initial assessments', *Text*, 18(2): 211–239.

Reder, P., Duncan, S. and Gray, M. (1993) *Beyond Blame: Child Abuse Tragedies Revisited*, London: Routledge.

Rimmon-Kenan, S. (1983) *Narrative Fiction: Contemporary Poetics*, London: Methuen.

Rowe, J. and Lambert, L. (1973) *Children Who Wait: A Study of Children Needing Substitute Parents*, London: BAAF.

Rustin, M. (2005) 'Conceptual analysis of critical moments in Victoria Climbié's life', *Child and Family Social Work*, 10: 11–19.

Sacks, H. (1967) Mimeo lectures, quoted in M. Coulthard (1977) *An Introduction to Discourse Analysis*, London: Longman.

—— (1974) 'On the analysability of stories by children', in R. Turner (ed.) *Ethnomethodology*, Harmondsworth: Penguin.

—— (1992) *Lectures on Conversation*, ed. by Gail Jefferson, Oxford: Blackwell.

Sarangi, S. (1998a) 'Interprofessional case construction in social work: the evidential status of information and its reportability', *Text*, 18: 241–270.

—— (1998b) 'Institutional language', in J. Mey (ed.) *Concise Encyclopaedia of Pragmatics*, Amsterdam: Elsevier.

Sarangi, S. and Roberts, C. (eds) (1999) *Talk, Work and Institutional Order: Discourse in Medical, Mediation and Management Settings*, Berlin: Mouton de Gruyter.

Sarangi, S. and Slembrouck, S. (1996) *Language, Bureaucracy and Social Control*, London: Longman.

Sarangi S., Roberts C. and Moss, B. (2004) 'Presentation of self and symptoms in primary care consultations involving patients from non-English speaking backgrounds', *Communication and Medicine*, 1(2): 159–170.

Sarbin, T. and Kituse, J. (1994) 'A prologue to constructing the social', in T. Sarbin, and J. Kitsuse. (eds) *Constructing the Social*, London: Sage.

Schon, D. (1983) *The Reflective Practitioner: How Professionals Think in Action*, New York: Jossey Bass.

Schultz, E. (1990) *Dialogue at the Margins: Whorf, Bakhtin and Linguistic Relativity*, Madison: University of Wisconsin Press.

Scott, M. and Lyman, S. (1968) 'Accounts', *American Sociological Review*, 33: 46–62.

Seltzer, M., Kullberg, C., Olesen, S.P., and Ilmari, R. (2001) *Listening to the Welfare State*, Aldershot: Ashgate

Semin, G. and Manstead, A. (1983) *The Accountability of Conduct: A Social Psychological Analysis*, London: Academic Press.

Sheldon, B. (2001) 'The validity of evidence-based practice in social work: a reply to Stephen Webb', *British Journal of Social Work*, 31(6): 801–809.

Shotter, J. (1993) *Conversational Realities: Constructing Life through Language*, London: Sage.

Shuman, A. (1993) '"Get outa my face": entitlement and authoritative discourse', in J. Hill and J. Irvine (eds) *Responsibility and Evidence in Oral Discourse*, Cambridge: Cambridge University Press.

Silverman, D. (1987) *Communication and Medical Practice: Social Relations in the Clinic*, London: Sage.

—— (1997) *Discourses of Counselling: HIV Counselling as Social Interaction*, London: Sage.

Silverstein, M. (1993) 'Metapragmatic discourse and metapragmatic function', in J. Lucy (ed.) *Reflexive Language*, Cambridge: Cambridge University Press.

Simpson, C., Simpson, R., Power, K., Salter, A. and Williams, A. (1994) 'GPs' and Health Visitors' Participation in Child Protection Case Conferences', *Child Abuse Review*, 3: 211–230.

Slembrouck, S. (1992) 'The parliamentary Hansard "verbatim" report: the written construction of spoken discourse', *Language and Literature*, 1(2): 101–119.

—— (2003) 'Class and parenting in accounts of child protection – a discursive ethnography under construction', *Pragmatics*, 13: 1, 101–134.

—— (2004) 'Reflexivity and the research interview Habitus and social class in parents' accounts of children in public care', *Critical Discourse Studies*, 1(1): 91–112.

—— (2005) 'Discourse, critique and ethnography: class-oriented coding in accounts of child protection', *Language Sciences*, 27: 6: 619–650.

Slembrouck, S. and Hall, C. (2003) 'Caring but not coping: fashioning a legitimate parent identity', in C. Hall, K. Juhila, N. Parton and T. Poso (eds) *Constructing Clienthood in Social Work and Human Services: Interaction, Identities and Practices*, London, Jessica Kingsley.

Smith, D. (1993) *Texts, Facts and Femininity: Exploring the Relations of Ruling*, London: Routledge.

Spencer, J. (1988) 'The role of text in the processing of people in organisations', *Discourse Processes*, 11: 61–78.

—— (2001) 'Self-presentation and organisational processing in a human service agency', in J. Gubrium and J. Holstein (eds) *Institutional Selves: Troubled Identities in a Postmodern World*, Oxford: Oxford University Press.

Spratt, T. and Callan, J. (2004) 'Parents' views on social work interventions in child welfare cases', *British Journal of Social Work*, 34: 199–224.

Stenson, K. (1993) 'Social work discourse and the social work interview', *Economy and Society*, 22(2): 42–76.

Strong, P. (1979) *The Ceremonial Order of the Clinic: Parents, Doctors and Medical Bureaucracies*, London: Routledge.

Strong, P. and Dingwall, R. (1983) 'The limits of negotiation in formal organisations', in G.N. Gilbert and P. Abel (eds) *Accounts and Action*, Aldershot: Gower.

Sudnow, D. (1965) 'Normal crimes: sociological features of the penal code in a public defender office', *Social Problems*, 12(3): 255–276.

Tannen, D. (1986) 'Introducing constructed dialogue in Greek and American conversational and literary narrative', in F. Coulmas (ed.) *Direct and Indirect Speech*, Berlin: Mouton de Gruyter.

Tannen, D. and Wallat, C. (1987) 'Interactive frames and knowledge schemas in interaction', *Social Psychology Quarterly*, 50: 205–216.

Tapsell, L. (2000) 'Using applied conversation analysis to teach novice dieticians history taking skills', *Human Studies*, 23: 281–307.

Taylor, C. (2003) Narrating practice: reflective accounts and the textual construction of reality', *Journal of Advanced Nursing*, 42(3): 244–251.

Taylor, C. and White, S. (2000) *Practising Reflexivity in Health and Welfare: Making Knowledge*, Milton Keynes: Open University Press.

—— (2002) 'What works about what works? Fashion, fad and EBP', *Social Work and Social Sciences Review*, 10(1): 63–81.

Thoburn, J., Lewis, A. and Shemmings, D. (1995) *Paternalism or Partnership? Family Involvement in Child Protection*, London: HMSO.

Thorpe, D. and Bilson, A. (1998) 'From protection to concern: child protection careers without apologies', *Children and Society*, 12: 373–386.

Tice, K. (1998) *Tales of Wayward Girls and Immoral Women: Case Records and the Professionalisation of Social Work*, Urbana, IL: University of Illinois Press.

Todorov, T. (1977) *The Poetics of Prose*, Oxford, Blackwell.

Toulmin, S. (1958) *The Uses of Argument*, Cambridge: Cambridge University Press

Toynbee, P. (1999) *Guardian*, 18 January, p. 16.

Troyer, R. (1989) 'Are social problems and social movements the same things?', in J. Holstein and G. Miller (eds) *Perspectives on Social Problems*, Greenwich, CT: JAI Press.

Tunstill, J. and Aldgate, J. (2000) *Services for Children in Need: From Policy to Practice*, London: Stationery Office.

Urek, M. (2004) 'Making a case in social work: the construction of an unsuitable mother', paper presented at the DANASWAC seminar, Huddersfield University, April.

Walker, S., Shemmings, D. and Cleaver, H. (2005) *Write Enough: Pitfalls for Practitioners* (4). Online. Available: http://www.writeenough.org.uk/pitfalls_for_practitioners_4. htm (accessed 19 April 2005).

Watson, D.R. (1978) 'Categorisation, authorisation and blame: negotiation in conversation', *Sociology*, 12: 105–113.

Webb, S. (2001) 'Some considerations on the validity of evidence-based practice in social work', *British Journal of Social Work*, 31(1): 57–79.

Weed, L. (1971) *Medical Records, Medical Education and Patient Care*, Cleveland: Press of Case Western Reserve.

Wheeler, S. (ed.) (1969) *On Record: Files and Dossiers in American Life*, New York: Russell Sage Foundation.

White, H. (1980) 'The value of narrativity in the representation of reality', *Critical Inquiry*, 7: 5–27.

White, S. (1999) 'Examining the artfulness of "Risk Talk"', in A. Jokinen, K. Juhila and T. Poso (eds) *Constructing Social Work Practices*, Aldershot: Ashgate.

White, S. and Stancombe, J. (2003) *Clinical Judgement in the Health and Welfare Professions: Extending the Evidence Base*, Milton Keynes: Open University Press.

Whorf, B. (1956) [1940] 'Science and Linguistics', in J. Carroll (ed.) *Language, Thought and Reality: Selected Writings of Benjamin Lee Whorf*, Cambridge: MIT Press.

Widdicombe , S. and Wooffit, R. (1995) *The Language of Youth Subcultures: Social Identity in Action*, Hemel Hempstead: Harvester Wheatsheaf.

Wilkinson, J. (1999) 'Implementing reflective practice', *Nursing Standard*, 13 (21): 36–40.

Wilson. T. (1991) 'Social structure and the sequential organisation of interaction', in D. Boden and D.H. Zimmerman (eds) *Talk and Social Structure: Studies in Ethnomethodology and Conversation Analysis*, Cambridge: Polity Press.

Witkin, S. and Harrison, D. (2001) 'Whose evidence and for what purpose', *Social Work*, 46(4): 293–296.

Woolgar, S. (1988) *Science: The Very Idea*, London: Tavistock.

Woolgar, S. and Pawluch, D. (1985) 'Ontological gerrymandering', *Social Problems*, 32: 214–27.

Wortham, S. and Locher, M. (1996) 'Voicing on the news', *Text*, 16: 557–585.

Zimmerman, D. (1969) 'Record-keeping and the intake process in a public welfare agency', in S. Wheeler (ed.) *On Record: Files and Dossiers in American Life*, New York: Russell Sage Foundation.

Author index

Subject index

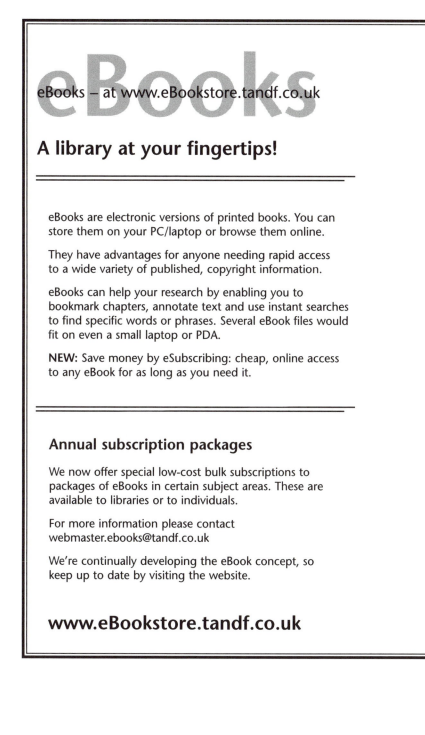